Without Prejudice?

An inspiring true story of a life-changing
liberation from a narcissist

Trish Valleys

Bombadil publishing

ISBN: 978-1-912354-07-8 (Paperback)
      978-1-912354-08-5 (e-book)

Any references to historical events, real people, or real places are used fictitiously. Names, characters, and places are products of the author's imagination.

Book design by Contentra Tecnologies Pvt. Ltd.

First printing edition 2021.

Publisher
Bombadil Publishing

'You're not a victim for sharing your story. You are a survivor setting the world on fire with your truth. And you never know who needs your light, your warmth and raging courage'

—Alex Elle

Contents

Illustrations

1. Love Letters?
2. Birthday Greetings
3. A New Threat
4. Connor's Cars
5. Christmas Greetings
6. Connor's 21st

Some final thoughts

Acknowledgements

Reviews

Foreword

Absolutely anyone can be a target of a narcissist. No one, regardless of gender, education, family background or career choice is immune to the charms and manipulation of a master narcissist. Trish's story is a painful yet revealing look into being locked under a narcissist's control and how it dismantles one's identity and self-worth.

Too often, victims of abuse are forced into an apologetic existence. They begin to believe what the narcissist says they are: weak, incapable, stupid, foolish, an embarrassment. The narcissist is so ashamed of themselves that they project it onto their victim. Only then can they attack their own shortcomings and dehumanise that same person they claim to love. At their core, narcissists are lonely and weak and deeply jealous of others who are successful and content. While a narcissist is incapable of loving anyone but themselves, they simultaneously harbour incredible self-doubt and low self-esteem and thrive off of conflict and deceit.

Trish has provided a rich and detailed account of the experiences of living with a narcissist. She shows us that while we can be broken, we can also be reborn. Trauma, grief and growth are all processes that put the human spirit on trial and Trish's life shows us that we can come out on the other side better, stronger and wiser. We are not who our abusers say we are. We are not broken, cracked, or ruined. We are strength and love and perseverance. We are brilliance, hope and peace.

Look to Trish's story as a guide for waking up from the nightmares and moving forward into the light. If you find yourself reflected in her words, realise that you are not alone.

Kristy Lee Dracker Hochenberger, LFD, MBA
Knowledge crowns those who seek her
Habere et dispertire

Kristy Lee Hochenberger is a doctoral student (ABD) of psychology at Capella University and a member of Psi Chi, the *International Honor Society in Psychology*. Her areas of expertise include child psychology and early education, narcissism and post-traumatic growth. A native of Queens, NY, she currently resides in upstate New York where she is an adjunct faculty member at *Syracuse University School of Information Studies* (iSchool) and University of the People.

Her accomplishments in the field of narcissism and abuse are already far-reaching and I began following her articles in *Psychology Today*, where she is recognised as a narcissism expert. It was an immense relief to find out that it wasn't me and I wasn't alone. At long last, I had an expert's thoughts as a lifeline and a way of moving myself forward.

Review by Dr Emma Katze

Written by a wise survivor, this little book will be of use to anyone who has experienced a bad relationship (or knows anyone who has). The book tells the story of how Trish Valleys broke free from a controlling domestic abuse perpetrator after many years of suffering. Trish's story includes issues that are rarely talked about: non-violent domestic abuse, abuse in small rural towns, the long battle of post-separation abuse, legal and economic abuse, the sexist responses that women still get from some professionals when they seek help, and how perpetrators only get away with much of their abuse through the (often unintentional) complicity of various systems and professionals. Throughout the book, Trish includes helpful advice to current survivors to help them achieve quicker and less expensive escapes to freedom.

Dr Emma Katz, Ph.D. Liverpool Hope University.

Emma Katz is a UK-based domestic violence researcher at Liverpool Hope University. Katz's definition of how coercive control affects children and young people has been cited in *The Guardian*, and is used by Welsh Women's Aid https://www.hope.ac.uk/si/dr-emma-katz.html.

Once more, I am grateful for all the work of Dr Katz and her team. It gives hope that eventually this form of non-domestic abuse will be given priority and the world will recognise the importance of supporting those who have suffered from it.

Introduction

I find introducing myself quite a challenge! Thinking of a short bio took longer than much of this book! I also realised that there is probably another book's worth of my life before my toxic relationship.

Work-wise I was pleased with myself in that I had been successful at everything I had tried my hand at, though I was of the mind that I wasn't sure what I wanted to be when I grew up! My natural talent at school was science and maths. Hence, I think my English teacher would be truly amazed to see my handiwork in this book. I had started out at work as a bank cashier and quickly became interested in financial planning and how it impacted people's lives. I retrained as a holistic financial and investment adviser and loved developing relationships with clients and planning for their futures. I still work with some of these people and can see the plans we put in place some thirty years ago coming to fruition. Amongst all this, I also worked as a contracts manager for my first husband's company and enjoyed the diversity and challenges of being very much part of a man's world of work at that time in steel fabrication. I think the two aspects of my work gave me insight into the workings of businesses and finance and how planning can be such a game-changer. All this was highly challenging at times and very busy. I loved the energy and activity and the buzz it gave me.

I was very young when I met and subsequently married my first husband. He was a widower with two daughters so I had the very special honour of a readymade family. About eighteen years later, I had a yearning for my own birth children and I went searching for the man who would deliver my dream. I met my second husband at a time when I was more concerned with my ticking body clock and desire for children, rather than properly evaluating the man himself and the quality of our relationship. Although having had such a wonderful first marriage, I was perhaps viewing life through rose-tinted spectacles. With this man, I realised my desire to have my own child and this will be the crowning joy in life until my dying day. However, almost without noticing in the first few years, I was on a descent into a world of abuse and control, and in the process losing my self-esteem and confidence. It was not until I was more than twenty years into our relationship that I became familiar with the term narcissism and some of the traits displayed by someone with those tendencies. I now believe that I was married to a narcissist as he displayed most of the traits that define those with a narcissistic personality disorder:

- Grandiosity. An exaggerated sense of self-importance
- Excessive need for admiration
- Superficial and exploitative relationships
- Lack of empathy

- Identity disturbance
- Difficulty with attachment and dependency
- Chronic feelings of emptiness and boredom
- Vulnerability to life transitions

Whether he was or not, it was most definitely an abusive and controlling relationship and psychologically very damaging to me.

Our relationship also followed the classic cycle of extreme narcissistic abuse and included the three stages: idealisation, devaluing and discarding. I have only recently learnt these terms, as I didn't think of our marriage as domestic abuse until it was nearly over. I was convinced it was more to do with my own failings as a wife and mother.

There were many times in twenty-five years when I didn't call the police or report the behaviours; I now realise this was from a sense of shame and guilt at my failure to measure up to what my husband wanted in our marriage. There was also a part of me that wanted to protect our son and perpetuate the projection of a happy family. The reality is that he also suffered in a very emotionally abusive situation.

I wrote this book in order to time tag the events and take a reflective look at how my life changed. It has allowed me to appreciate the good times, understand the bad times and validate myself.

I have spent many hours working with a therapist and initially this was done in secret and paid for privately. Yet again, I felt enormous guilt and regarded myself as the creator of my fragile mental health. I also felt that if there was any mention of mental health problems on my national health records, it would possibly stand in my way for future employment prospects. Both of these factors hampered the development of my emotional intelligence.

That said, I've learnt a lot about myself and how to appreciate my resilience over the years it has taken me to gain my freedom, and I want to share this so that others can take shortcuts.

Now I feel I have largely recovered from this experience, and have some thoughts and ideas which may be of help to others who are in similar situations. This is my small contribution to opening up and shining a light on the dark world of domestic abuse and coercive control in a relationship. I hope it provides help for those who are in broken relationships at whatever stage. This could be either the avoidance, extraction or recovery stage.

**Dedicated to INCA my first triad on the recovery road
and my incantations**

I spread good

I embrace life

I share feelings & spread laughter

I influence & inspire others

I help others

Sociable
Aware
Relaxed
Influential
Generous

INCA

Warm, firm, not a tense body
Flowing soft & graceful
Stand grounded, rounded shoulders, relaxed hands
Seeing my reflection sparkling in the eyes of those I'm with

I'm master of my own destiny
I enjoy a powerful feeling of being genuine
I bring out the best in people with the best of myself
I give people purpose
I draw people to me

I embrace people

I'm curious to know them

I'm generous

I'm influential

I'm lovable

I'm competent

I'm assertive

I have beauty

Why this book **?**

I have been trying to find cases and insights to read and found very little which is written first hand. Maybe, like me, many people who have suffered abuse, particularly when part of it is coercive control and financial abuse, are embarrassed or ashamed of it. Possibly they are still recovering, or in a better place and not wanting to revisit such difficult memories. I wanted to read articles by others with similar experiences, in order to get a handle on how they coped and survived. Most important for me were some ideas and self help for survivors of this kind of control on how to regain their lives. As I didn't find much of any help, I decided to journal my thoughts and experiences, in the hope that some of what I experienced can be of support to others.

I'm not sure whether, for me, writing this is a way of putting it all in its place - in the past - and enabling me to manage my new life going forward. Part of it may be that I hope that some of what I experienced will resonate with others who are caught in the same situation. I have tried to reflect on some of the major events of my relationship and appreciate the learning. I have noted a couple of my key findings below the relevant sections, which may or may not mean anything to you.

It has shown me all the learning I have done and everything I have managed to achieve. I am a survivor and do not intend to sit down and fade away anytime soon. After years I have managed to take charge of my life and I want to offer my support to those who are still struggling at the hands of an abuser. I am accountable and recognise all that I have done and lived through and am able to take charge of my future destiny.

I hope the message, that there is light at the end of some long tunnels, gets through in the words. We can all become masters of our own futures if we use the learnings from these abusive relationships to create new futures for ourselves and live our dreams.

Above all, I hope to help those who are stuck in a bad situation to take action and move to a better place!

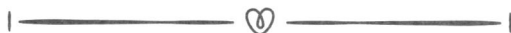

So here goes……. And if you're wondering about the title 'Without Prejudice'? I decided on this thanks to the abuser who is now NOT in my life! Every communication, whether by text, email, or handwritten, he marked 'Without Prejudice'. Whether it was a belief that if he stated that at the outset, he could then say what he liked to me, I'm not sure. I thought it appropriate to write this book and use the same phrase for its title.

I was thirty-five and, after a rebellious teenage stage, had had a successful start to my career, a fabulous love life, fun and travel. The main reason for this joy was my first husband Graham, who was a widower and his two daughters, Sarah and Beth. Sadly, for them, their Mum died very young from cancer. I was hooked on this readymade family. Graham was a fun, young at heart, hard-working, adventurous and spirited entrepreneur, with his own business and a large extended family. He was a generous warm-hearted man. His daughters were wonderful, loving and engaging. Life was very family-orientated and I remember how warm it made me feel to be a part of such a life. Graham was quite traditional in home-life matters (he never cooked a meal or washed up), and he was very supportive and encouraging. If I voiced any desire to do something, even if it had been to go to the moon, he would hug me and say 'go girl'. He especially liked it if it involved a work project and me asserting my equality in a meeting full of men! He was a massive fan of equality for women in the workplace. He gave me great confidence that I could achieve whatever I put my mind to. It wasn't a perfect relationship, but it was based on love, mutual respect and compassion – all important values for me.

Graham was a lot older than me and so there is not so much of an age gap between my stepdaughters and me. This presented some difficulties at first but was the best of life experiences. To this day, the girls and I are best of friends and their children are friends with my son. I even recently became a great granny!

Despite this happiness, my body clock suddenly started ticking loudly and I was obsessed with having birth children before time ran out for me. Sadly, Graham declined all enticements to father my children! Being older, he was not inclined to turn the clock back to the baby stage. Our marriage ended in an amicable divorce and we remained friends until he died a few years later. He was overjoyed for me when I had a son, who he met several times. Maybe he somehow knew that any children he fathered with me would end up with the same loss and grief his girls had suffered with the loss of their Mum. He would never have wanted that to happen.

So there I was, looking for a willing father and in a hurry! Looking back, I also had an unnerving amount of self-confidence and assuredness as to what I wanted and how to get it. Much of this was the legacy of Graham and the girls.

Fast forward twenty-five years and I wonder what happened and how? I'm not even a shadow of that woman.

I have tried to recount my story and put some of my reflections and the lessons I learnt under each section, in the hope that those who follow may avoid some of the pain.

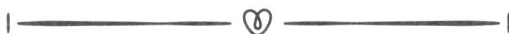

——————— ♡ ———————

How it all started ?

I was in my mid-thirties, divorced and had been pretty successful in my career when I met William. We met on a social night out, and many of my usual instinctive checks were swept aside in the excitement of a new relationship.

- *Learnings are to take stock of what I have achieved and where I am.*
- *What do I want my life to look like as a Mum?*
- *What do I want for my career in addition to being a Mum?*
- *Always have a plan for the short, medium and long term.*
- *Treat each new relationship with a suitable amount of caution, whether that is a romantic or work situation.*

William was in his late thirties and had never been married. I ignored that warning signal of 'Why hadn't he been snapped up?' as he told me he had a couple of long-term relationships. Later, I was to find out that long-term was a couple of months.

Whenever we went out on dates, he always took me out of our area, again a warning signal that I chose to ignore, thinking he wanted to have as much time as just the two of us, making new memories.

He used to take me out in his mother's car. Naively, and ignoring the warning sign again, I thought he just wanted to impress as it was a Mercedes and, in his view, better than the car he owned.

Going dutch on our dates, I thought that was the modern independent way. He told me he was short of cash, as he had bought a new business, which included a retail premises.

The relationship progressed and I moved in with him after around a year. Someone once told me, 'you never know someone until you live with them'. I think this is so true. Before we lived together, we both had our own homes and work lives. We only spent evenings or weekends together, it was easy to only see what I wanted to see of his world and ignore the bits I wasn't so keen on. At different stages of our lives, we can choose to see things through rose-coloured glasses. I now realise this is not the way to enter into a long-term relationship.

- *Ask yourself why they don't introduce you to their friends and family?*
- *Intimate dates are ok but what is day-to-day life going to look like?*
- *What are the different views of their local community? Does everyone speak well of your partner?*
- *Ask questions about them to others and try and get different perspectives on your relationship!*
- *Keep reminding yourself to trust your gut and any messages it is giving you!*

Babies and marriage

We had had a few conversations about babies and having our own family and decided we would try. I was in my mid-30's at this time and he was in his late 30's. As it is for so many, it was more difficult than expected and so after twelve months we moved onto fertility help and IVF. By that time, I was helping with the running of his retail business to a great extent, as well as continuing my business. Despite medical advice to take things easier, it was never a consideration that I should stop work. Indeed, it had transpired that much of the funds for the business purchase had been 'loaned' to William from friends and family, and needed repaying.

At that time, no free help for IVF was available in our area on the NHS. As it was me 'failing' to conceive, our relationship had dropped to a blame game at times. One of these was me and my age and being nearly too old at thirty-eight! Because of this, I felt it was my responsibility to pay the bills for the treatment. William was one of several children and therefore he and his family thought there couldn't be a fertility issue on his side of the family. Once again consultants advised me this wasn't the truth, but I chose to ignore that. Because I had the funds and wanted a baby, I funded this incredibly stressful treatment. My parents also helped and I cashed in some savings to support the cycles of IVF. Success came for us in the third cycle and the greatest experience of my life, our son, Connor, was born in 1999. This was four years after William and I had met. For me, it was the greatest of my dreams come true. William, I now realise, was excited to be able to claim a father's bragging rights. However, I now believe that began one of the worst emotions a possible narcissist feels – envy. Regrettably, I spent many years explaining to our son that his Dad's acts of jealousy were his expressions of love. How did I get that so wrong? From my own perspective, I couldn't understand any parent not feeling an all-encompassing love for their children, let alone be jealous of them.

- *Ask yourself if it's good to take up with a partner with this level of debt.*

- *On any major financial decisions, make it a discussion and a joint plan, don't just assume the burden.*
- *Ask yourself, what is my partner doing to support me, not blame me, in this process?*
- *Never confuse your child with the incorrect labelling of emotions. Children's intuition identifies emotions. Help them to know which emotions they are and let your children know they can trust their gut.*

For a short while, William was the doting father and insisted on getting married and doing the right thing by his son. (He later admitted that the only reason for marrying was to ensure that Connor had William's surname, not mine.) Naming our child was a bit problematic as William was adamantly against anything I suggested and would only agree to use names he chose which were William's father's names. Nothing I could say would change his view. It was just another action in stripping me of any recognition, self-confidence and voice in this world.

Our wedding was a well-kept secret on William's terms. He didn't want me to have a stone in my ring as I might scratch the baby with it; he didn't want a big, showy wedding as his brother was marrying later in the year and that was enough fuss; he didn't want to invite any of our family and friends; and so we had just a quiet registry office affair with two witnesses. This passed me by at the time. A wedding of any sort was a minor event compared to me in the euphoric state of being a new Mum who thought she'd never give birth and would miss motherhood. In the grand scheme of life and miracle births, marriage wasn't so important to me. However, these were a few little flags I missed at the time. Now I reflect and see that this is all part of the way this kind of abusive relationship develops, insidiously and gradually.

- *Run everything by a trusted friend to check their take on your decisions. Get other perspectives to make sure yours aren't becoming too narrowly focussed.*
- *If you haven't got someone you can talk to, go and tell your doctor or another professional. Keep a narrative going with them so they have a baseline assessment of you and can advise if they see changes happening. Why does anyone who is in love want to keep a marriage quiet?*

We returned to our home next to the business premises and settled into more of a routine for a while. As I was self-employed and William spent many days away from home, I was very busy with a baby, running William's business and trying to keep up with my own work. Part of my own work involved going to see clients in the evenings, so I soon found myself working seven days and evenings a week. This was somewhat hampered by the fact that William failed to come home to look after Connor when I had made appointments with clients. If I commented on this lack of support, I was reminded that I only had one child to look after whereas his Mum had managed six children. At the time, I accepted this as William's justification for not babysitting his son. As a new Mum, this didn't help my confidence and in order to become a better Mum (I believed), I started to reduce my own business and time spent with the clients. I was gradually falling into the trap of trying to be a supermom as well as juggle work and finances.

- *Ask where your partner is spending his or her time and for some help co-parenting and sharing the load, both with the work and finances.*
- *Don't take on board any guilt and share ownership of any problems.*
- *Keep a realistic view of what you can achieve every day and get your partner to share the load as equally as possible.*

The move to the country

Before Connor was twelve months old, William came home one day announcing he wanted to move us out into the country. I said we were in the country and a village. He argued the case that he wanted to move Connor further from the main road so he couldn't get harmed. (Our house was on a B road just before a T-junction and with a gated garden.) I wasn't overly concerned about the traffic problem. I asked where he thought and he took me to see a piece of open ground of a few acres with no house or accommodation. I asked where we would live and what did he want this much ground for? William decided he wanted to farm, an ambition which came out of the blue as I had never heard him talk about this before. His plan was to live in an old rented bungalow two miles away. I asked what I was going to do with my career, as I had no plans to be a farmer or live in an old damp bungalow while Connor was growing up. William suggested we try and get planning permission on the ground for a house and then we would have a proper farm. I agreed to this plan on the sole condition that, once we had achieved the target of a house and built the farm, we could sell it and do something else. I didn't want me or Connor spending the rest of our lives in the hills, working 24/7 for very little reward. William's family was also surprised at his sudden desire to farm. When his father had been diagnosed as terminally ill and was making his will a few years before, William specifically told his family that he didn't want a farm. Had William expressed the desire to be a farmer then he would have inherited the family farm, as is the traditional patriarchal way in rural parts. Still I didn't see the flags which were waving on a fairly regular basis. Instead, I heard the promises made by William that the farming wouldn't take much time and that he would generate a good income by trading four-wheel drive vehicles as well, so we would be financially ok, and I could be a stay-at-home Mum. That was a great carrot for me.

I had done some research and concluded that it would be very difficult to produce much of an income on such a small piece of ground and was concerned as to how we would afford any kind of life up in the hills. However, on the up side I was a country girl and there was a pull towards living a natural, healthy country life and rearing our own food.

These thoughts gave me the idea for the farm business. What about organic produce and in particular poultry? The organic movement was still in its infancy at the time and it wasn't possible to buy organic produce from supermarkets very easily. Poultry doesn't graze grass, so the fact that we only had a small amount didn't matter. We could put up significant amounts of housing for poultry on a few acres and buy-in all the food. With that idea in mind, I agreed to attend the auction for the sale of the land and borrowed a sizable amount of money from my parents to put down the 10% deposit required on the night, if we were successful.

- *Look carefully at anything which is isolating, whether that is where you are living, your ability to maintain and build links with friends and not just family, as well as work and social opportunities.*
- *Stay visible to society!*
- *A partner who loves and respects you as an individual will also understand these individual needs as being important, not just tending to their needs.*

Life building the family and home

We were successful and so the next major lifestyle change happened in my life. We were now the lucky owners of some derelict acres of grassland with various rough patches and some grass, not many gates and a few strands of wire as fencing! We called it Pinewood. William's mother had also been in contact with a neighbour who had a bungalow next to her which we rented. We sold the house and business premises in the village. One fortunate friendship I made was with the buyer who needed help for a few weeks with her daily book-keeping tasks. It's eighteen years on and I'm still involved and that is one relationship that kept me sane and in touch with the wider world and gave me a reason to get down out of the hills several times a week. It also became a base for me to re-start my business and become independent since applying to divorce William.

- *Keep hold of friendships and do whatever you can to go and visit or get them to visit you regularly.*
- *Insist on taking young children to nursery or playgroup at least once a week. It is a vital social interaction for you as well as them.*
- *Get a part-time job for a few hours per week. It may not be the best paid but it is rich in self-worth and confidence-boosting factors.*

One of the positives of owning the land was that I could finally have a horse. These noble stoic creatures have enormously helped me over the years. They have helped me carry all sorts of baggage and helped me get rid of it! They have been a silent non-judgmental support for many miles of my journey. In addition to their loyal and stoic characters, they have connected me to some amazing friends. Ironically, my first horse ever was a rescue mare. I discovered her in the back of a lorry at a sale and managed to get her for a few quid cash. The problem with my having a mare on a farm was that William decided she had to earn her keep by producing foals which he could sell. (His fervour to sell wasn't restricted to just the foals. Sometimes I would find my horse had been sold. My car and even Connor's pet dog disappeared one day, when William had a cash offer.) Later on, after William had rejected organic farming, he bought more foals and unbacked horses. I then had the job of training and starting the young horses so that he could sell them for profit. Alongside other small farm livestock and animals, this is an extremely labour-intensive way of making a living. Although it was lovely to spend time with the horses, what was originally just a hobby and pastime became a burdensome chore.

So my riding was restricted to fine weather when my mare wasn't too heavily in foal or with one suckling. This usually meant a plod round the lanes or on the open hill if we ever had enough time to get there.

It is easy to dwell on the negative in this book, but actually making this record has encouraged me to remember many things and so many happy times as well. Connor played a massive part in this joy, along with the horses and people I met because of them. It leads me to the conclusion that I have had challenges in life and that has given me some amazing experiences and lots of learning opportunities. Some of them I might never want to repeat, and at least I can now recognise them and steer a different course accordingly!

We moved to the little bungalow and life was busy. Connor was becoming an active inquisitive toddler and I had many happy times showing him the world around us. We began repairs to the fences of the fields we now owned and bought our first few sheep and cows. At the same time, I was researching and putting together a business plan for organic poultry production and presenting this to the local authority with an application for a farmhouse and dwelling. I didn't miss the people and social aspect of life at first as it was very busy just keeping up with all the home and family and also 7 days a week jobs on the farm! There was virtually no time for my own business and the internet was poor, so it became more awkward to stay in touch with clients, family and friends. On top of all this, I had a hankering for a brother or sister for Connor. William wasn't so interested and said it was down to me to fund any more IVF. We tried one cycle unsuccessfully and I was advised to consider counselling and potentially a donor egg. After several missed appointments to go for counselling William told me he had been discussing this with his family and they didn't think we should proceed, rather we should leave things to happen naturally. I think at that time I was more upset that this was the end of my potential to give birth to a sibling for Connor. I didn't really reflect on the fact that this major life decision William had taken was in discussion with his family and not me. He just delivered the verdict and I didn't spend time wondering why his family came in front of his wife and son in the talking and planning. Once again, I was emotionally quite fragile and possibly not in a place to see the logic. I did try and get this message across to William and wanted to talk about the decision, but he seemed to have moved on and expected me to do the same. I did the same as I did not want to miss the joys of the child we already had by spending my life grieving for what was not to be. I did write William a letter and described my feelings and thoughts about the way he had made the decision and what it made me feel like. I found the note returned under my pillow and the subject was never brought up again.

- *Get professional help, such as talking to someone if there are major events in your life.*
- *Talk to the business and financial planners, the bank manager. Don't keep secrets! If something is bothering you and you can't have a proper and meaningful discussion with your partner, seek out professionals to help. Talking it over gets the problem out and you don't take sole responsibility for the problem. This allows you to maintain perspective on situations and your self-esteem. Don't let the darker moments snuff out the light from all the joyful ones. There will be moments of peace and happiness. Spend a few minutes each night before bed thinking about and appreciating all the good bits of your day. If necessary write a long list of all your daily wins.*

I threw a lot of energy into developing an organic poultry business for the farm and applying for planning permission to build a house. The authorities deemed it necessary for us to demonstrate three years' business trading before granting permission, and in the interim allowed us a mobile home. This presented us with an opportunity to build a mobile log home which, if we were successful with planning, we could subsequently holiday-let. The planners liked it as a concept and so we got to build and live in a log cabin. It was like being on holiday after the old damp bungalow, a little small and all in together, but hey ho, we had the great outdoor space as well. Fortunately, and rarely in the UK, we had amazing spring and summer weather the year we spent in the cabin. Connor and friends spent long warm days outside and camped in tents and a teepee we had made in the field. I had no garden or vegetable patch but planted seeds everywhere I could. Every day Connor went out and collected enough veg of different sorts to make a meal. I will always remember the courgettes: they flourished so well we had them with every meal in every conceivable form!

We started off with our poultry and for a year the new adventure and project went well. I began to think it might not be so bad being up the hill and 'out of it'. Connor started school, which took me into daily contact with other parents, and very quickly I was enlisted as chair of governors. I was there until Connor had nearly finished high school. I like to think it is because everyone wanted me to help support the school but sometimes wonder if it was because I needed their help and support.

- *Get involved in any way you can when the children are at school, even if that's getting there five minutes early to talk to other Mums. Make an effort to get to fetes, parents' evening and plays. It is a free support and variety for you.*

Life on a rural farm

Having a log cabin to holiday-let strengthened my business plan, so the planning went smoothly and we started to build our own house. For once, William was home a great deal as he was labouring and supervising the build. As with everything, there was little we agreed on at times, which led to a few walls being built and then taken down again as William had different ideas to me. It took a good many months but eventually, we had a house. As it neared completion, it became obvious William didn't want to fund things like the kitchen, the white goods, a television, etc. By this time I had withdrawn most of my savings so I chose to get a loan; it was made clear to me that I would be making the repayments alone, but we finished the house and had a home.

Once again, there were a peaceful few months as we settled into Pinewood and worked on the farm. William started to disappear more frequently once the house was built, often without explanation or reason. Originally, he had promised that the farm work would not take up much of the day and that he would help supplement the income by doing vehicle repairs and sales from the farm. This failed to materialize and it seemed that his time away from the farm was spent at his mother's farm or local livestock markets. Over time, I learnt that these efforts to make us more economically viable as a farm business were nothing of the sort: they were just time away for William who was increasingly withdrawing from us as a family and also from work and the business.

In what seemed like no time at all, William came home with a desire to buy more land two miles away, next to his mother's farm. Seemingly, this was where he really wanted to be and not at Pinewood. He suggested that as I had been successful with a planning application once, perhaps I could try again and we could go and live there. I was very annoyed and concerned as this was not what we had planned or agreed to when we bought the first piece of ground. Farming was not making any money and I could not see that more land was going to make a viable business. Indeed we were only staying afloat with the holiday-let income and the profit from my business. (My work had shrunk by that time to some book-keeping and VAT and payroll, as I didn't get to go out and see clients anymore.) William was inflexible and adamant. His family was also quite surprised. As I referred to earlier, they confirmed that he had not been even remotely interested in farming when his father asked him if he wanted the home farm. Now he was doing anything he could to get land and live right next door.

In the interim, I had inherited two small amounts of money and so eventually this was put towards the purchase of the land. Prior to signing this over, William and I specifically agreed to sell the first farm as soon as possible and concentrate our efforts on only one piece of ground. He had reassured me that the piece of land would not take much management and he would still be at the home farm in the main. I held onto the hope that this new venture would renew William's interest in both the family and the farm. This was not to be and of course, he disappeared most days and the farming at our home was largely left to me. This meant very long days and very lonely work. I was now plucking and dressing poultry and then attending farmers' markets at weekends to sell the produce on my own. Christmas was becoming a nightmare as we had hundreds of turkeys and geese to get to customers. Although a number of the elderly relatives came and helped plucking, it was down to me to organise sales, delivery, payment and packing. I found it incredibly stressful being responsible for all those Christmas dinners and if a delivery went astray, how it would ruin a big day. For several years, I was exhausted by the time Christmas Day dawned, so much so it was hard to enjoy time with Connor as I usually felt ill. One year I had pneumonia and have never felt so poorly.

I was successful in getting planning permission for another holiday log cabin at our farm and also one at the other piece of ground. I spent most of my inheritances on the second cabin at Pinewood as I calculated this would help the income. It was a slow process but lettings increased and I was once again keeping our heads above water. Combined with the other jobs I was doing, it made life a bit easier again for a short while.

- *Even if you have a business together, maintain some form of bank account in your own name and regularly check your joint credit scores to make sure you are fully aware of any problems. Open a separate bill-paying account and make sure you each pay in or have the money paid in from the business to cover the outgoings. Don't take on debt, credit cards or any other finance and shoulder that burden alone. All outgoings for the household and family should be shared between you.*

Peace didn't last long, as William soon decided not to complete the required organic scheme maintenance and didn't want to stay in the scheme. We received support payments for this provided we kept to our contract. As this wasn't complied with, we found ourselves faced with withdrawal of the organic support. This entailed a reclaim of five years' payments and the last of my inheritance went to repay this.

I was starting to feel frustrated and weary that whatever we did, there was never enough income. Living an 'idyllic' country lifestyle was proving very expensive and tiring. In addition, William disappeared every day to his mother's farm. I found this irritating as it didn't help our situation but it didn't worry William. His mother's farm was very small and she was still very active, so I couldn't understand why this was a daily part of life. I also began to worry about moving over to a piece of land right next door as I could imagine that we would never see William.

- *Don't do this! Talk to whoever you owe money to and get a JOINT repayment plan! Do not put yourself in the position of being solely responsible for paying joint debts.*
- *Do not let embarrassment or shame get in the way of a completely open and frank talk with your solicitor or whoever is preparing your financial claim. Ensure they know what kind of person they have in opposition and have full facts of debts. Even if they are in your sole name, they have been incurred by the two of you.*

Appreciating the rural life

I don't want anyone reading this to feel that my life was completely without joy and good times. Living where we did was a fantastic environment. We were fortunate to be living on a hill with amazing panoramic views of the river and valley below us. Whatever the weather, there was always something to see which gave me pleasure, even if it was watching a storm coming towards us! I loved nature, the wildlife, the dark skies at night and the feeling of space. This environment helped me escape for a few minutes every day. Looking back now I am reminded of all that I achieved in that place. Sometimes it's easy to forget that just simple things, like a walk through the fields, or watching new born lambs playing in the sun, would bring joy to my world. That and being lucky enough to work at home meant I spent many more hours with Connor unlike many parents who have to go out to work.

- *Look for the positives in your life and make the most of them. If you spend just a few minutes each day smiling it will lift your spirits and improve your resilience. Take time to appreciate all the good things no matter how small. If you can get to look at the clouds every day, it will help lighten your mood and put a smile on your face*

The road to divorce

Slowly but surely our marriage was crumbling as we seemed unable to find any common ground or interests. If I mentioned holidays, William would state that he didn't intend to travel past the end of the drive. I gave up on the idea of a family holiday and took Connor alone for a week away. When we got home, I found my vegetable garden and paddock next to the house had been dug up, and William had partially erected a wall and drive in their place. This felt to me like a punishment for going away. I gradually lost interest in gardening and growing our own veg as any of these hobbies were being spoilt over time by William's behaviour. Nearly everything I attempted or did was becoming the object of a daily insult. Gradually, I lost confidence in myself and my ability to succeed in even the most menial tasks. I stopped finding joy in anything except Connor's life and achievements. I was determined he would have more confidence than his Mum and encouraged and supported him in every way I could think. This actually made William worse. I am not sure to this day whether it was jealousy of Connor or spite for me. I didn't really need to know, I just needed to escape from this seemingly happy place that had turned into a nightmare. I tried talking to William and reasoning with him. This got no response, so I tried confronting him about getting a proper paying income and having the farm as a hobby. The original promises of vehicle sales and repairs had dropped off the radar. I wanted to develop a plan of action and see where we could change our lives and pull the happiness and family life back together and all go in the same direction. William wasn't a willing partner in any discussion and used to walk out, and later he would leave me notes and instructions on the kitchen table. So when the talking didn't get any results I tried the same tactic and wrote to him. While I always read and tried my best with his letters, the same didn't appear to be true of William. More than once, I tried writing a letter to him in the hope that it was his preferred style of communication. My letters were always put (apparently unopened) back in the drawer in the farm office and out of sight. To this day, I do not know if he ever read one. So communication was a one-way street as far as letters were concerned.

- *Every day, list even the smallest of your achievements and keep adding to them. Read them regularly and stand in front of the mirror and smile at yourself. Remind yourself of all the great things you have achieved. Find self-help groups and learn coping strategies if you're trying to make the relationship work. Seek professional help through your GP and talk to support groups online. They will be able to advise you and help you if the situation is becoming abusive. You don't always recognise it as abuse because it is so much a part of your normal day!*

Reading back over this reminds me that I am emotionally in a vastly different place today and so I do make this book sound a little as if it was a very black and white situation and there was a definite plan! This totally wasn't the case. Virtually, every day was a negotiation of who was doing what, our precarious financial situation and what were we going to do. Clearly, things didn't get settled and I was getting more and more depressed. After some months of William telling me it was my problem, I did embark on various self-development courses to improve my attitude and communications. I mastered some of these skills and used them to help overcome and reframe some of my thoughts into more positive feelings. It did work and I felt for a while that I had resolved the issues between us by developing a better way of communicating. Along the way, I had made friends with the wife of the self-development trainer and she, Jess, was a good support. She also bought a horse and kept it at the farm with us. Horse livery was something we had taken on at the farm in a bid to increase our income. We now had one or two people liverying their horses with us or keeping their young unbacked horses on our fields. Although it increased the workload, I enjoyed getting to spend time with horses, even if they did belong to other people. If work allowed, Jess and I would go hacking out around the local lanes every week and I felt my life was improving. She became quite a major pillar of my support system. Yet the workload and the financial debt mountain were still growing. I took on several more ideas and plans to increase our income but was finding it all exhausting and unsustainable.

Years were drifting past and with each year was a bigger mountain of work and debt. I made many attempts to talk to William to resolve issues but he did not want to engage. I started to feel very frustrated and angry and finally, in 2014, I went to see a solicitor and filed for divorce. Reflecting on this I wonder if I could have improved my communication with William, but over the twenty years together we both seemed to have changed completely. One thing that really troubled me was that it was becoming increasingly clear that my values were a world apart from William's. I think I was so focussed on making our family a unit which worked together, I hadn't noticed that there were grass-root flaws which would never allow that to happen.

Well, for better or worse, (and believe me some days I think it is worse!), I went ahead and issued the petition. It was the summer holidays and I had forewarned Connor of the impending divorce. He was bewildered and a bit anxious and, to be honest, I was feeling much the same. So a summer holiday passed without me being able to support our son in a time of need. Strangely, this is one of the times I look back on with regret. Every day I say sorry for all the things that I have got wrong in life, ask forgiveness, express gratitude and give myself love. I find this helps me recover from the traumas and become a confident human again. All the years I spent doing my very best to shield Connor from the abuse and the hurt and I still feel guilty over this stage.

- *When you go to a solicitor ask them to fight as hard as they can for all you are entitled to. Do not accept a legal adviser who wants you to be pragmatic. Definitely, do not go to your solicitor and put forward ideas which you believe will be the best for your partner! Do not believe that settling for little or nothing will get you out of the abusive controlling situation any quicker. Remember, it's not just the financial abuse, it's coercive control, so why would they want to stop? Making an offer to an abuser lets them know you are still bending to their will and in their control. Sadly, although these are criminal acts, very few legal professionals or judges recognise and see this big picture. Inadvertently, with all the pragmatism and offers and waiting, they play the abuser's game, while you pay for the costs of it. Admit debts to the conversation, even if they are in your name. Make sure you explain how they relate as joint debts. If a spouse has fraudulently obtained credit or loans in your name, contact the card or loan company and explain and ask them to investigate.*

The petition

Soon after William received the petition mysterious problems started happening. I had bought myself a car, much to William's disgust and criticism. About nine times over the next few weeks I had flat tyres when I went to drive off in the mornings. It was really odd as I had parked my car in the same place and used the driveway for fourteen years without a problem. Eventually, after spending a small fortune on new tyres I managed to get insurance against future flat tyres which still had tread on, and free replacements. I left a copy of this insurance on the kitchen table and the problem cleared up - magically I had no more flats.

The next mystery problem was that various items of furniture and clothing and household goods were rearranging themselves overnight. Sometimes I found things outside or a room had been trashed or items were missing. In the past, I had had periods of sleep walking and William blamed me for these incidents. He told me I was losing it (my mind?) and that I must be doing it in my sleep. I was seriously worried about this as I had no recollection of anything and also could not find any evidence that I had been sleepwalking (no dirty feet, etc). To be certain, I bought a 'Fitbit' with a sleep tracker. I didn't tell William about this and initially only wore it in bed. Oddly, the next time the house was rearranged it showed me that I had been sleeping soundly and hadn't taken any steps at all. I was relieved but a bit unnerved by what was happening. Clearly, William was the perpetrator as there was no one else in the house and I really didn't understand his reasoning for trying to make me think it was me.

- *Don't keep this behaviour hidden and say nothing. Some people don't report this because they have no proof. This isn't necessary. Go to the police and make full reports. Let the police do their job and investigate how this was happening and who is responsible, not shoulder the worry yourself. It will also provide a useful log of events if you need to go for a restraining order. Explain you believe this to be abuse and request an officer with specialist training andknowledge.*

I am finding it harder to write each day as I get closer to the present. I thought I couldn't face any more abuse and fatigue before I petitioned for divorce, but the current systems and legal route to get free from a coercive controller are much bigger challenges. Or perhaps I was supposed to be so relieved to escape that I ran and hid and asked for nothing financially. Five years and nine months after first applying for divorce, of which three years are post-divorce, I have little to show for it. It has cost me countless amounts in legal support and worst of all is I'm still not free from the control or received the financial settlement that was originally agreed over three years ago.

When William first received the petition, he seemed fairly reasonable and suggested that we didn't sell the house until the following year when Connor had completed his GCSE exams. His rationale for this was that it would be more stable and enable Connor to achieve. I had my doubts as to whether this was in Connor's best interests because up until that point, William had always criticised Connor's ability and education as a whole. He continuously disrupted Connor's homework and study with requests for help with the livestock. Looking back, I now realise that this was really to give William an opportunity to start removing equipment, livestock and other assets and cash so that the financial settlement would be less for me.

Mediation

I suggested that maybe there was room for mediation and getting some counselling to see if there was any way forward other than divorce. We went along to a session with a mediator (after two missed appointments by William). For over an hour, I barely got to say a word and listened to a continuous denigration of my abilities by William. He clearly thought he had found the ideal person to listen to him rant. I found it quite disturbing that this person who was supposed to be a mediator, seemingly just sat there and at no time attempted to tell William he had had his say and perhaps I would like to say something. However, the mediator (apparently an authorised and trained counsellor) did conclude at the end of the hour that, 'Mr Fielding you have talked about your marriage as a business proposition and not a relationship. You have not expressed any emotion and solely concern yourself with the financial viability of a business'. I asked the counsellor if there was anything she could suggest that would help and received no response. However, this is a procedure that has to be followed before applying to the court for a divorce. It has to be demonstrated that efforts have been made to resolve the issues by both parties. I am sure there are cases where this format works and rescues a marriage, but clearly this wasn't suited to our 'business'. I got the distinct impression the mediator was happy to sign this one off as a 'no resolution other than divorce' case. Which is exactly what she did.

- *Don't accept any delay. There is never a right time to divorce, just get it done sooner! This is merely an opportunity for an abuser to exercise his power and control. It only extends the pain and misery. Mediation has to be considered first when applying for the divorce. Make sure you request a specialist mediator who is well-informed on issues of control and abuse. If you're not happy with the services of professionals let them know! As above, many people are not yet trained in recognising the very subtle signs of abuse. The little things are the very important instances which, if ignored or not understood, can make it feel it is a very broken and unsupportive system which currently exists in the world of divorce.*

As William suggested we delayed, so as early as possible after Connor's exam the following year, I asked for the house and farm to go on the market, and for William to make an agreement with me over the finances, Connor's future and living arrangements. A couple of months later Connor got the exam results he needed to get a place at college. As we were in such a rural area with no transport links, it meant that he would be living away during the term time. This was a relief for me in some ways as it was hard keeping the house and family 'normal' routines when in fact all I wanted was to be free of this situation. I never wanted to escape being a mother to Connor but I did want to stop the pretence that our family life was okay with William. I was exhausted and it was all I could do to cope with William's behaviour, while shielding Connor from it as much as possible. I believed that we could make an agreement between ourselves and it would be easier and quicker and less costly for all if we did so. As we had been together twenty years, and much of the value of our assets had been built together, it seemed a simple enough task to agree. How wrong I was and how little I now feel I knew William and his family. Over the years, I had given all of his siblings and his mother considerable support and help and been part of the family in a very active way. Once the divorce was announced, all family contact was cut immediately. Even when I answered telephone calls from any of them, I was spoken to as if I was a complete stranger. Not one person ever asked me if there was anything they could do or offer a chat or support.

- *Stay calm. This is about their inability to communicate and not yours! Ensure you inform all those around you of your situation. Schools and colleges will keep an eye on your children and support them if necessary. Ensure estate agents and conveyancers involved in property sales are fully conversant with ensuring equality for both parties and consult jointly at all times. I found to my detriment that conversations held separately with William and me were always distorted and unhelpful.*

Friends and divorce

Around this time, my friend, Jess, also announced problems with her marriage and intention to divorce. I did my best to support her and it seemed a fairly minor indiscretion on her husband's part which had caused their split. I liked both of them and worked with her husband from time to time. However, I didn't want to be between them at such a time. I explained to her husband that I would be dropping our work and contact and supporting his wife, which he understood. Jess continued to come to see her horse and for a while, we were closer than ever as we supported each other on our divorce journeys. The money she paid for the keep of her horse also helped at a time when our income was exceptionally low.

- *Yes, help friends and also step back and try and look at your own situation without the emotion attached. You can help friends because you aren't emotionally entangled. Do the same for your own situation and look objectively with a stranger's eyes.*

A particularly difficult time for me was trying to negotiate the financial settlement with William. He had grown to believe (or so he told me) that all our assets were his and that I hadn't contributed to anything; any assets he had in his own name weren't to be included in the settlement. I was weary and anxious to get away as my mental health was suffering from all the mind games William was playing. Jess also started suggesting that I reduce my claim for finances. I felt this was a bit odd and told her so as I had just helped her get a very good financial settlement during her divorce, which had been completed in a couple of months.

Another thing that bothered me was the couple of times I had noticed that William had some information regarding fairly trivial matters not relating directly to the divorce. One day he said something about one such matter and an alarm bell rang in my head. How had he got the information? Thinking about it, there were three possible people who could have passed it on. Our son, an elderly friend and Jess. I decided to see who it might be and gave them each a different piece of unimportant information and waited. I was dismayed to find that the information I gave to Jess found its way to William. I made excuses for how this could have happened and passed on three more scraps of information to the three likely suspects. The result was the same. Forewarned, I was then careful with every word I said, but it was hurtful and I was really saddened by the fact that I no longer felt I had someone who I could trust to support me. I'm not normally mentally slow but really couldn't understand why Jess was betraying me. However, it was soon lambing time on the farm and the reasons started to become clearer. Jess wanted to come over and stay. She had time off from work and so we could have 'girl time' and go riding. She wanted to stay in the log cabin rather than the house. I mistook this for her feeling uncomfortable with William and me because we now argued regularly. Connor being away at college made room for overt aggressiveness and arguing on most days. As William continually refused to make a financial agreement, other than one in which I walked away with nothing, it was getting very heated.

Anyway, Jess stayed in the cabin and I was in the spare bedroom in the house William was out tending to lamb duties at the other farm. For some reason, one night I woke as I heard his car come home around midnight. I heard it stop at the top of our drive and not down by the house as usual. Some 5 hours later, I was woken by the dog barking as William came into the house and went swiftly upstairs to his bedroom Clearly, he had spent the 5 hours somewhere and I believed it to be with Jess. My mind was racing with what to do and whether to confront them and ask what was going on. I had no evidence that he had been to the log cabin and not just been attending pregnant sheep in our fields, so I decided to wait and see what other signs might show up. I was also, by this time, half-minded to believe that if William were keen to start a new relationship, he might release me and make an agreement. How wrong I was and I'd known him for twenty plus years!

As I hadn't any evidence to confront them, I resolved to watch and wait and in the meantime only give information to Jess that I wanted transmitted to William. At the same time, I felt I had been betrayed by someone who I trusted and had confidec in. There was nothing obvious, except that Connor commented that his Dad had taken him to Jess' house one day. I didn't ask anything just noted it.

- *Be very careful of who you trust. It is easy when you are going through such ordeals as an abusive relationship, to rely on friends who may not be what they seem.*
- *Be wary of secrets too. Many abusers groom their prey by getting their victims to keep secrets. Help your children to understand that secrets are not a good thing.*

Soon afterwards, a mutual friend of our family was holding an event in Comb our local town, and he invited us along to the show. There were plenty of places so I asked Jess if she wanted to come. She wasn't really interested and so declined. A few days later she sent an email saying that William had invited her and she wanted to let me know that she would come along with us, only if I understood that it wasn't a date I found this truly amazing. Why would I think such a thing? To be honest, I was pas caring what either of them did really, or whether or not they were dating each other.

Had I chosen to simply walk away, she would have potentially walked into the farm and I now began to understand her reasons for trying to convince me to reduce my financial claim in order to get a settlement.

I decided to make light of everything and to carry on as if nothing was amiss The afternoon before the event we arranged to go for a ride and afterwards go on to the event in Comb together.

The day dawned and William informed me he would be taking Connor to the event. I wasn't too bothered and thought that Jess and I could go a little early and have a snack and drink before the show. We rode out and then Jess announced she was going home to shower and change. She lived a round trip of 40 miles away, so had often brought her clothes and had a shower and changed at the farm after riding. What was different on this occasion? Why hadn't she brought her clothes as before and showered at the farm? Anyway, Jess said she would meet me there. I carried on and the time came to meet her and she wasn't to be seen at the place we had chosen. She wasn't answering her phone either and the doors to the event had already opened. I went in to reserve spaces for us. There was no sign of her, or Connor and William and then, just as the doors were closing, they came in. Connor first, looking anxious and headed my way as soon as he saw me and took the seat next to me. Jess and William both had drinks in their hands and so it was obvious they had met up beforehand. They took up seats behind us and I was desperately holding it together for Connor, but felt completely let down and upset. It wasn't just for myself, but for the fact that William was trying to put Connor in the position of condoning his actions with Jess and making him choose which parent he was supporting. Fortunately, the event was interesting and spared me the embarrassment of having to turn around and make any small talk with William or my rapidly becoming ex-friend.

By this time, I was weary of the whole situation and when I accidentally caught them smooching on the lawn of the log cabin, I just walked away. A few hours after this incident I had an email from Jess, accusing me of being unfriendly and she didn't know what she had done to be treated so badly. Finally, something snapped and I felt so angry. This was becoming a more frequent emotion and I hated it and the way it left me feeling. I decided the best course of action was to phone her and record myself doing so, in order to check that I kept my temper. Jess picked up the phone, heard my voice and hung up straight away. I phoned back and this time spoke to the answering machine. I said I had decided that we weren't friends anymore as I needed space to get myself sorted. I asked her to ask William to move her horse as soon as possible so that she had no reason to visit the farm. I put down the phone and replayed my recording to ensure I hadn't raised my voice or been impolite. Satisfied, I left home to go to work and consequently went out of mobile signal, as the work was in the depths of the hills. Later that evening, when I came back into signal, a cascade of texts greeted me. Two were from one of my 'friend's' other boyfriends, who had texted to tell me how ridiculous I was and how upsetting it was for Jess. The second was about the horse and how removing him would leave me with no friends! I did feel like responding that with this kind of friend I didn't need enemies!

Interestingly, the last text came from William, who also told me I was destroying the best friendship I had ever had and that I didn't know how lucky I was to have such a friend. Even more interesting was his comment that he hadn't slept with her in the log cabin! Really? I hadn't mentioned anything to do with William or divorce, and I certainly hadn't mentioned anything about them sleeping together in the log cabin when I made my announcement of ceasing our friendship. I merely blamed it on me being too distracted with life! For better or worse, I decided not to respond to any of them. For once I didn't feel the need to justify myself. Jess' horse was moved a few days later and William continued for several months to tell me how stupid I had been over my decision. Oddly, it did make my decision-making over our finances a little easier, as I wasn't constantly worrying whether I was being fair.

- *If you have a gut feeling over these things, act on it quickly and decisively. If you get it wrong and it's a genuine friend they will stick by you and will understand. They will not send you letters of blame and will not make you feel you're the one in the wrong. Always trust your gut, it won't let you down. Sometimes it may take you a while to figure out what the message is that it's trying to give you but stick with it. It may just be getting you to notice incongruences! Real friends won't keep secrets from you!*

Court hearings and delays

After the ending of the friendship, I found I was more able to concentrate on my own needs. The financial settlement was complicated by the fact that we had two farm businesses and one had originally been owned three ways with William's mother. This all sounds very glamorous and fruitful, but please don't be deluded. Farming and agriculture is an incredibly demanding occupation, a seven-day week job with many night as well as day shifts. The hourly rate works out in the pennies. Small farms make no money at all and are only sustainable with an income stream from outside, usually done by women. I was typical of that setup and our little farm businesses were kept afloat mainly as a result of my other work.

I made various representations to William via my solicitor based on what I believed was fair. One night, about a month before we were due to attend a court hearing to decide the finances, William agreed on a settlement figure. It was fairly low as I had agreed not to pursue a share of the woodland his father had given him and also that I would pay off all the loans and debts in my name. I was exhausted at the time and just wanted an end to the marriage and a sale of the farm so that I could move on. William wrote out the agreement and I typed it up. He suggested that if I disinstructed my solicitor, his solicitor could then draw up the agreement for us and send it to court. All would then be settled and we wouldn't need to attend court. I did as William suggested the next day and we sent our agreement to his solicitor.

Life became painful that afternoon as I tripped over one of the farm collie's puppies and broke my ankle. I tried to ignore it but it got worse so I ended up at A&E having an x-ray and a support boot. The next day our agreement arrived for checking and signing. I checked and sent back a couple of spelling errors and agreed to sign. William was slower and it was getting very close to the court date. I asked him to sort it so that we didn't have to go to court and he agreed, knowing that the court date was on Thursday at 9.30 am. He told me that he was going to the Storeham livestock market on Wednesday morning and that he would go to his solicitor's and sign as well and get him to let the court know. At noon on Wednesday, I had the telephone call from William who was in his solicitor's office. He advised me that his solicitor had told him he had agreed too much of a settlement and so he had changed his mind and wasn't signing the agreement. I don't know why I had believed William would honour his agreement. I was angry, frightened and now without legal representation. I stayed up the whole night preparing myself to act in person. It was quite scary walking into the courtroom (well hobbling) and trying to conduct my own case. The judge was far from pleased that no preparation had been done. I explained that this was a bit last minute as we had had an agreement, but it was a lead balloon. She adjourned and instructed me to get various papers ready for a new date. I was relieved that I would now get a bit more time and hoped desperately that we would get the same judge who now knew that it had been William's deceit that had led to this case.

Up until now we hadn't sold anything and I had no money to fight this battle, so I decided to continue representing myself. I did what I thought was sensible and took a friend as my 'McKenzie friend' to the next court appearance. I had provided the evidence to the court of William's Mum's retirement from the one partnership. This meant that it was now a two-way split not a three-way split in the ground we owned. However, William was still hell-bent on trying to get the land for himself and not prepared to consider a fifty per cent pay out to me. He kept insisting, wrongly, that his Mum had not been bought out of the partnership and that together they held two-thirds of the ground and I was only a third owner. The judge concluded that there would be a trial on the issue and instructed me to get a court 'bundle' ready. In the interim, William's Mum, who had already declared that she knew she was no longer a partner, had a stroke and was rendered unable to attend court to state her case. Much to William's dismay, his sister and brother, who were attorneys for their mother, decided against pursuing the matter further, at the time.

As I wasn't to know that William's Mum would be withdrawing due to her stroke, I had visited a solicitor for some advice on producing a court bundle. The solicitor listened to me as part of a free consultation and then declared that he believed he should act for me, not just help with the court bundle. I must admit I was tired and stressed with the whole idea so having someone help sounded like a good idea at the time. In addition to the strain of court proceedings, William was vociferous about the fact that he believed me to be responsible for his Mum's stroke. Medical evidence would defy this, but William preferred to blame me for causing her so much anxiety because I was divorcing her son. I had always done my utmost for the family and liked his Mum. We had spoken briefly about the divorce and breakdown of the marriage and while she was sad about the situation she had never given me any indication that she was stressed about it. Nevertheless, it was another metaphorical swipe at my mental health and self-esteem.

- **Follow your instinct and don't disinstruct solicitors or do anything else based on what your partner says. They are just laying the groundwork for the next manipulation. Stay strong and for as long as you believe someone is doing their utmost for you, keep them instructed. Additionally, put them on a fixed price or agreement for each piece of work. Sadly, many solicitors are motivated by the size of the settlement and determine their fees accordingly. This is a completely corrupt and distorted way of conducting business and does not represent value for money. Stay firm and ensure you get value for money from your legal advisers. If all else fails and you cannot afford a solicitor, you can decide to represent yourself. This can be an advantage as the judge is obliged to give you time and is more lenient over the process. You can take a friend into court with** you, a McKenzie friend, who can support and can help take notes and hand you papers. Remember, you know your own story very well and so it is not so hard to present it to a judge. Contact me if you need support.

Yet more delay

It was another year, two more court hearings, hours of talks and gigabytes of emails between solicitors before William finally agreed over the finances. However, in that time I had started to suffer dramatically from the stress of still being under his control and living in the same house. I was desperate to get an agreement and consequently made some very rash decisions over finance, which weren't helped by solicitors advising me to be 'pragmatic' all the time. My solicitor didn't seem to be aware that my situation had all the hallmarks of financial abuse and coercive control. Among other things, I agreed to pay all the household bills so that Connor had some kind of home, and even though William was living there, he didn't want to contribute towards anything except some firewood. Even his solicitor was surprised (by the look on his face) at William's lack of concern for his son. Additionally, I agreed that William could exclude a piece of woodland worth tens of thousands from the joint assets and also reduce his assets by a substantial figure as he said it was to repay a loan to his brother. Regrettably, I was so anxious for the whole farce to end, I didn't ask my solicitor to get evidence of this loan. I do not know when William lent the money to his brother and I never asked to see the loan agreement. The concept of us splitting everything half each didn't work in my case. This was because William wouldn't agree to pay half towards the debts and loans, which although they were joint, had been put in my name. This was despite me agreeing to allow one hundred percent to William for the purported loan to his brother! I also agreed to make applications to remove the agricultural tie from our property and if I was successful I would split the uplift in value equally with William. As I eventually got another £..,000 that was a gift of half the increase for William. Consequently, I agreed to a financial remedy order of about 30% of our assets, which is pragmatic to say the least! The benefit of hindsight has shown me how not to deal with finances when I am in a highly emotional state. I settled for the sake of a quick exit and also because I felt guilty at that time that I was the one who had failed to keep the marriage going and was leaving. Contrary to this, William, who had received some windfall shares from a joint insurance bond (because he was first named on the policy), did not split the value equally with me.

- *If you get into this situation, do not be 'pragmatic'. It will not be good enough for an abuser and you will lose financially and emotionally. Ensure every asset and every liability is entered and go for at least 50%. If you are caring for children or paying the household bills go for more to cover these costs. Don't forget to look at pensions you both have and make sure you split the benefits equally. Make sure you claim half the value of items like windfall shares.*

Trying to feel safe

All these incidents were coming thick and fast, all at the same time not one after the other. Life at Pinewood was very heated and argumentative most days and even when Connor was home from college it became difficult to pretend we had a normal life. In fact, only recently, Connor remarked on the rows and atmosphere back then. Nothing escapes children, so it's best to be honest and upfront with them, and of course in an appropriate form for the age of your children. Unfortunately, Connor had the rows to suffer when he was home though at least that was only every few weeks. However, he did not fail to notice the lock on my spare bedroom door. I dismissed it as trivia, but I am sure he didn't believe me. His father always behaved well when Connor was at home. (That way he could always state that it was my imagination.)

While Connor was away, William had made various attempts to sexually assault me. Initially, I had moved into the spare room but he had made a couple of attempts to get in bed with me, so I decided it was safer to put a lock on the door. Being locked in my room made me feel safer and when the inevitable insults started I could just go to bed. During our marriage, I had been compliant to whatever his needs and desires were, believing that was my role. At times, I had questioned why there was no consideration for my needs and desires but this didn't warrant a response. Now I cringed at the very thought of him coming near me. Inevitably, one night, the unthinkable happened. I was absolutely sound asleep. The locked door made me feel safer and looking back, I'm sure that is why I was so peacefully asleep. All I remember was waking when I felt him trying to enter me from behind. I screamed in my absolute panic. I scrambled away, first to the bathroom and then downstairs and outside in the clothes I had on. I raced for the sanctuary of my car and drove up onto the open hill. I was in a terrible panic and couldn't fathom how he had picked the lock and got in and how I hadn't heard and woken! Why did he think he could do such a thing, or even enter my locked bedroom when we had been divorced six months earlier? I didn't know where to go or what to do; I knew I was too embarrassed to tell anyone. I slept in the car and returned the next morning when it was daylight as for some reason that made me feel it was safe! Looking back, I can't really see what my reasoning was. He had already gone so it was safe. I returned to my room and dressed and went to my day's work, all the time wondering what was best to do and how to ensure it didn't happen again. My first action was to buy a better lock for the door which I installed straightaway.

Since the days when the furniture was being rearranged at night and William started accusing me of anger problems and losing my sanity, I had been considering seeing a counsellor. I researched specialists and went to see one. This I did privately, once again to try and make sure there was nothing showing on my medical records which could affect my credibility in my professional work in the future. It was a means of self-help and getting advice and coping strategies. Still being in the same house as my ex-husband was having a great emotional and psychological impact, and sessions with my counsellor helped.

After sorting the lock, I arranged a session.

The next night all was quiet and no attempts were made to test the new lock, but it was a sleepless one for me. The next day, I saw some elderly friends and decided to tell them about the incident. They were concerned and pressed me to report it to the police. There had been many occasions before when I had considered calling the police and had always decided against it as I was very worried about the impact on Connor. I had carried on in silence. However, now that Connor was older and William's abuse was becoming more extreme, I thought it would be safer to call. I must have picked up the phone a hundred times before I finally rang the non-emergency helpline to make the report. The police officer was patient and helpful and gave me advice on staying safe and encouraged me to call immediately if there were any other incidents. He also gave me a safe word to use. Later that afternoon, a local policeman phoned me to say he had received the report and said he wanted to come and interview me at home. I felt that this would be very risky if William were to arrive when the police were there and also that it would put me in danger of repercussions after they left. He asked me several questions as to how I could manage and I explained about the better lock and that I had been advised to ring 999 and report anything further. No one confirmed whether they had spoken to William and to be honest I was rapidly going off the idea. I was feeling concerned about the consequences if William was spoken to. I was starting to feel I should have just kept quiet and hoped it wouldn't happen again. I felt totally unsafe and alone. Reflecting on this, I am now even more disconcerted that the police did not even find me a safe place to interview me and support me. I believe there is still an attitude that as I had been his wife in the past, it wasn't really a rape situation. In the end, I got a WiFi security camera for inside the house and a wildlife camera for outside, as well as a better lock for the bedroom door. Both cameras were quite revealing as to who was coming upstairs when I wasn't at home and also the wild William who put nails behind the wheel of my car so that a puncture resulted when I reversed over it. Sadly, I had the stock answer from the police a few times – 'it's a civil matter'.

- *Never keep quiet. Tell the police and tell your friends. Keep telling the police. Even though domestic abuse is recognised as a crime, I believe that many don't think of it that way because these people were once partners and you had consensual sex. Keep telling them even if they don't want to hear. Keep telling them it is coercive control and remind them it is a crime. Don't be silent or believe it is your fault. It's not and if you stay silent, you feed the abuser's habit. This is one of the tunnels where there is light at the end which is easily reached. Keep flicking the switch!*

Surrendering things

A couple of weeks after I made the report, a policeman and woman came to call and ask us to surrender our shotguns and firearms and also our certificates. Part of the rural life on a farm is the need to deal with vermin, especially the foxes who loved an organic poultry supper. We both shared guns in order to be able to manage vermin control. William wasn't at home so they telephoned him to ask him to come to Pinewood. He was not pleased about the circumstances of their visit and was childishly ranting and raving as usual. The policeman explained that allegations of attempted rape had been made against him and they were obliged to recover the shotguns or firearms unless an alternative solution could be found. This propelled William to near apoplexy and his verbal belittling of me was incredible. I was shaky but feeling that if anything got out of hand the police would be able to protect me. The policewoman was remarkably unsympathetic and said nothing to calm the situation. In fact, she said nothing at all. On later reflection, I wonder if she was just there as part of the lip service to equality. The only solution the policeman proposed was if William moved out to his mother's he could take his shotgun and firearm to her farm and gun cabinet and relinquish the keys to the cabinet here at home. I could then keep my gun at home. William was cursing and definitely not going to move anywhere. There was no other option offered and so we were obliged to surrender our guns and certificates. The policeman said that our guns would be returned once we had sold the farm and moved away from each other. William's expletives went on and on while he handed over the guns and the policeman's final comment was, 'I know what it's like mate, I've been divorced twice'. That remark was another blow to my confidence. Clearly, the police supporting William's behaviour made him feel entirely justified as to what a stupid c...t I was. He was malevolent and of course had just had his ego stroked and supported, and therefore was completely convinced of being justified in speaking to me the way he did. For a moment, I felt completely broken and it was hard to think logically and decide what to do next. I was tearful and feeling vulnerable. As the police were leaving, so did I. I felt it was best to be out of the way while William calmed down and I drove out behind the police car to find a friend for a cuppa in safety. My friend came with me when I returned to Pinewood and William was all sweetness and light. He didn't mention the earlier events and surprisingly only brought it up at the height of later arguments. I have been trying to get my gun returned since we sold the farm in October 2017. Unfortunately, though I have had a medical report vouching for my sanity and suitability, William gave the police a story about being worried about my temper and that the finances weren't sorted so I might harm him if I was allowed my gun back. I understand the predicament of the police with issues like this, but really am very frustrated at the fact that William can use statements like this to continue his control of yet another part of my life. It is sometimes hard to take a step forward because all these chains are still padlocked. I now realise that wanting my gun back is just so that I can make a choice of my own. I no longer need it as I no longer need to do any vermin control. However, I want to be the one who decides when to sell it and what to do with it, rather than when William allows it. To some degree, it will be when William allows, because my gun will only be returned once William confirms that he and I have no contact with each other. While I have already given the police this reassurance, they do not get the same response from William. No doubt it's his last little power play and control of me.

- *Remind the police and any other professionals of equality and ask them if they are trained in how to deal with coercive control. Ask them if they recognise that this is what is happening to them? They have to deal with very difficult situations such as these, but it can be done with an attitude of equality to both parties.*

William's tactics of verbal abuse increased several-fold after this. Although, to my knowledge, he had never met my first husband on a one-to-one basis, William started telling me he had had several conversations with him. One he particularly liked to tell me about was that my first husband had regretted our divorce and had wished that he had slit my throat instead. Ludicrous though it seems now, I was almost convinced at times that this was the truth. I had seriously lost faith in myself and was at a very low ebb. Now that William was using the other men in my life to back up his view of me, I really felt I was an utter failure. William nastily told me that slitting my throat was probably the best thing. I was very frightened and worried that my end was near, either at the hands of William or just my heart giving out with the stress of it all. I kept asking myself, what did I do to deserve such loathing.

- *Keep a handle on reality and make sure you aren't convincing yourself something is true when it blatantly is not. Don't let the abuser's distorted view of you convince you that it is fact. Hang in there and look at the facts of each situation, not what the abuser wants you to believe.*

The learnings from this are that I realised how low my confidence and self-esteem were. Time to get more help – big style! I couldn't afford to increase my private counselling so I went to the GP for help. This came in tablet form and I could not manage more than a week on the anti-depressants he gave me. They no doubt work for many, but I hated the drowsy feeling and that I couldn't care less. Presumably, these work on the theory that I couldn't be depressed about nothing and I certainly thought of nothing that week. I was also troubled by the idea that it would be on my medical record if in the future I went for a job or asked for my guns back. I decided it was best to get some more counselling privately and was lucky enough to find someone fairly local. I still see this counsellor as I have found a new, positive, addiction: I am addicted to recovering myself and restoring my self-confidence and esteem and with it, my mental health. He has helped me look at all the events and learn new coping strategies while forgiving and loving myself and accepting that I'm not perfect. It has been a revealing journey through a mental maze of anger, sadness and guilt and grief. I'm not at my destination yet, but I am enjoying this journey and discovering my strengths and skills, which were buried for twenty-five years!

- *It is natural to grieve for what has gone and you don't have to blame yourself or struggle with these emotions alone. See your GP for some guidance and talk therapy. Love yourself and be kind to yourself! Every day spend a little time appreciating yourself and all that you have.*

Illustrations

Trish,

I don't think there's anything clever about sending me letters of (solicitors) asking for money just because you have some now. (.....................)

Just let's meet up and sort this lat bit of money out. You can now afford to pay your dues!

I hope you don't think going back to court will be a bed of roses for you.

Whatever

William x

Illustration 1: *This is an illustration of the sort of 'love letters' I received. You will note that spelling and grammar were not his strong points, only bullying! This was what I received when I thought the whole saga would finish and before I realised it was possibly a narcissist I was divorcing! We had just sold the house and some land remained to sell to complete the financial remedy order. One thing I have learnt since is, do not respond. Take away all oxygen! Then the abuser cannot re-enter your life. Do anything you can for yourself and your sanity and leave the pen or keyboard alone. Join me again to find out just how long it was before I learnt that one!*

Ye guess it is my responsibility now, and should be (-without prejudice). Seeing I bought the farm and all the livestock, and my mum and I bought the extra land, which was then stolen off her. Bit hard for mum to go to court and fight her corner with THE TRUTH when in a hospital bed and unable to speak! OUR responsibility was to give Connor a safe and happy childhood so BIG FAILURE there (and NOBODY will EVER be giving forgiveness for that) the poor kid, and his own words quote 'I couldn't stay at home dad' (seeing his dad being battered not nice) and he so hated Tinmouth (college) and all those hours with a shrink! But hey ho I'm alright jack in the sun. Thank god he's maanged to get a job and is now living wiht someone nice, he knows I'm always here for him even though the farm I bought for him has gone. Fine if you want ot share this email. Just make sure the police who came to the farm and witnessed you admitting to kill me, and listened to me, and made notes of the abuse and beatings what I told them. I had been subjected to, are also sharing. Best contact me via solicitors, if U must! I'm sure they would love a bit more of MY money, without prejudice I'm guessing your solicitor has found out what this means by now. Without prejudice. Sorry 2 hear Bobby the dog mum bought for Connor has died, (I hope Connor had substantial money from Bobby's stud fees, as was your plan)? I've bought Connor another if he wants it. And I hope Connor can have the vaccination soon as the S/E seems to have high nos of the Coron thing. Wx

Illustration 2: *Little loving epistle sent on my birthday in 2021. Months after all was finally finished, it does not appear finished in his head. Admittedly, I had sent some final papers to him for the farm a few weeks before. They had come to me in error as he had obviously forgotten to change the contact details. After sending them to him, I had forgotten to block his email address. This was the response. I have now blocked the email address. Maybe I have to resign myself to little quips like this on high days and holidays. I'm still thinking what is best to do. It no longer worries and frightens me so much, but I do not want my life touched in anyway by this man in the future.*

Trish, ...

I don't think all the correspondence back & forth is getting anywhere ....

Best get some one to mediate to see if we can sort things without court? Because there is no way you will get away without paying your dues ie aforementioned payments owed to me on my letter of 20.11.20 ...

Then perhaps we can do a deal on the land, ... Remembering that it's mostly scrub not a pony paddock ...

Whoever, Whatever

William x

Illustration 3: *This was one of the enticing threats to try and get me to deal directly with a man who believed every asset of ours should belong to him. It was very costly but I decided to let solicitors deal with him. They had a very difficult time as they were also unused to having what I term a narcissist manipulating them, but at least I only got a few threats!*

> *The £1500 car I let Connor have, he had an accident and it's extremely damaged. So he is going to keep it. I've asked him for £500 to cover SOME OF MY LOSS.*
>
> *(been as you insisted on paying for half of his first card as you did not want me to be the golden parent).*
>
> *Perhaps you can find the £500 (out of the £ ..K you took,) don't see why I should loose both ways around.*

Illustration 4: *The context of this little note was that Connor's first car had failed its MOT. He had the car as a 17th birthday present and it was a cheap and cheerful Clio which was low-cost to insure and low CCs. William had bought the car at auction and then taken twice the value of the car as payment out of our joint farm account. (This was what he refers to above as me wanting to be the golden parent.) He also gave Connor a Land Rover, which he had owned for years, which was about 20 years old and a non-runner. I was really touched by this until I saw that William had taken a sizable payment (about twice its value) out of our joint account to pay himself for the 'gift'. The little Clio failed its MOT a year later so William gave Connor another cheap old car as a replacement. This was not worth £1500 and William bought it at auction for a third of the price. Unfortunately, Connor aquaplaned on a very wet night on his way up our lane and crashed into a neighbour's fence. Connor didn't tell either of us about the incident. Instead, he got friends to tow him out and took the car to a pal's where they repaired it. This car had done 150,000 miles before Connor owned it and was well-worn. There was damage, but Connor did his level best to put things right. He asked his Dad to help repair the neighbour's fence, which William refused to do and I stepped in and paid a local fencer the £75 to repair. Connor worked off this debt by way of housework and other chores. I was absolutely astonished that William put the price of a very old car above our son. Not once did he enquire if Connor was ok and unhurt. I felt sick to my core that William put money in front of his child. He then started asking Connor to pay for the car as he had damaged it. I have never seen my son so stressed. I was so worried knowing what pressure he was under from this man who was actually his Dad! We went to the cash machine and withdrew the money and paid William what he had asked. As you can guess, by now I was getting the message that money meant more to William than anything else.*

Trish WITHOUT PREJUDICE

I haven't sent your mum a Christmas card, so i'll leave it to you to give her the good news. Her daughter has 'finally managed to achieve something in her life'.... rob me and my family of my property and 10's of 1000's of our money - chucked in the gutter with as many 'good people - friends you let down and disregarded, along the way.

Ho, but you kept the best ones - like - your clever best friends (you know) the couple, one who pretends to be a Christian and the other gave you such good advice that we only managed to WASTE £40k on solicitors (I must write and thank them) that should have been Connor's inheritance. Last but not least your friend who sold you the bargain car for £7k now worth £3k. I expect your mum will come to the same conclusion as me ....
'WITH FRIENDS LIKE THAT WHO NEEDS ENEMIES?

Illustration 5: *This was the Christmas message I got the year that Connor and I flew abroad to spend Christmas with my family. A wonderful time which we talk about with many happy memories to this day. This little message had been put in my handbag and William rang me as we boarded the flight to let me know it was there. For a few moments, until I read it, I was touched that he had thought to pack a surprise Christmas card for me. How wrong I was! On reaching my Mum's house, I discovered that he had sent a ranting letter to my Mum as well. I have never seen the letter and nor do I know the content. My Mum and the family never discussed it or responded to it. I was glad Connor and I were in the safest and most loving of homes that year.*

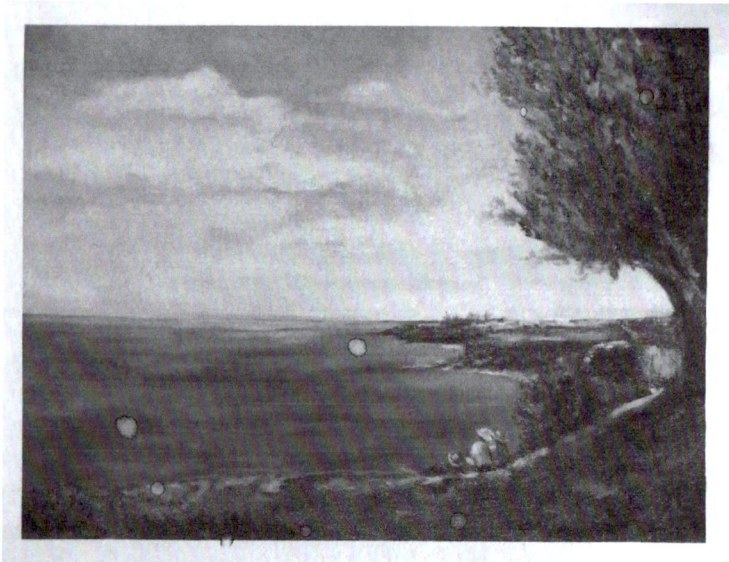

The first scan picture

Those cherry red lips when you were born!

A month like a puckered up dog's bottom in George's Marvellous Medicine

The morning Santa left your first pony

Pulling you on a plastic bag behind the quad sledging

Going to get the Harry Potter book in XXXX on your birthday!

Trekking to Nepal with a humanitarian heart

Fundraising & Tallship Sailing

Waiter in Chief at The XXXXXX

Mousse XXX & Tiramisu

Business Class Flight Birthday Cake!

Your college tutor singing if his daughter brought you home he'd be delighted!

Box of love you gave me on Mother's Day

Winning sports day obstacle race at primary school with your friend XXXX

Running up XXX XXX with your dog and your hair dyed pink for charity

Family Xmas in the USA!

Winning Best Baby at XXXXXX

Sardines on the beach at Fuengirola

XXXXXXXXX 1st Play at school

Waterslides into the field on your birthday!

First Wood Tractor

Happy Birthday XXXX!

I send all my love to you as you celebrate your 21st Birthday
May more of your dreams come true.
Our love holds us together each and every day
It doesn't matter the distance. we will always find a way
I want to thank you deeply for giving so much to me
I am so proud to have you in my life. Our bond will forever be
There have been so many joyous moments so far and reducing to 21 was a hard choice
21 wonderful memories for 21 great years

All my love.
Mum

xxx

Illustration 6: *I recently wrote this for Connor's 21st*

The equine assistance

The horses we had on the farm had become more and more important and gave me peace and tranquillity in some very stressful times. I learnt a great deal about how just spending time with the horses lifted my mood. Brushing them or just sitting beside them in the field and reading a book, all helped. I used to do regular sessions for my own mental health and well-being as well as offering sessions of equine-assisted development to anyone who wanted to come and unload their burdens of life and free themselves. All of this can be done silently and goes on internally, but it is amazing how good you feel after spending half an hour unloading your burden. It is something I really recommend as it is all about communication but not about words. It is a way of shedding the load of guilt, self-deprecation and worry. At the same time, I was doing some exercises and online courses in emotional intelligence. Gradually, over time, these two therapies helped me to begin rebuilding myself and help the stronger, calmer, more confident self-reappear. A year into the divorce proceedings and I felt strong enough to give up smoking and the self-development work and the horses helped with that too. It was almost like a soothing conversation going on in my head when I was with the horses. One day I was looking at my cigarette packet when a voice popped in and said 'you can do it'. I wasn't really focussed or thinking about smoking or giving up and as I reached for my next fix, I just had a thought of I'll have one in a minute. Five minutes later, I realised it had worked and that was the start. I just kept thinking in a minute and soon enough it was an hour then a morning and soon a whole day! I couldn't believe how easy it was to keep saying that to myself and it's now five years! Occasionally, I think about a cigarette and have to remind myself I don't smoke. It was this that gave me the start and I gradually began to think about being a survivor and the longer life I was possibly now going to live. I had been at a very low point and wondering if I had the strength and stamina to go through the divorce. I turned my phrase around and started looking forward and now say, 'I'll have my life forward in one more minute'. These tiny steps help me to manage my negative thoughts around never being free of this man and have pushed me forward. Some days it is a tiny step and sideways not forward, but it's never backward.

- *Find horses to be with, even if it's just a walk round the local stables or riding for the disabled. Go and groom or stroke or just lean over the fence and share your thoughts with them. You don't need words. The horses are remarkably able to take your burden and quietly ditch it for you. Give yourself a target which distracts you from just the end of the divorce road. Don't wait for it to be over before you plan exciting and new challenges in your life. Take small steps. Set SMART goals and break them down into small steps. If every day you take that small step you will congratulate yourself for achieving every day. This helps your confidence. If you try a huge leap and miss you will destroy yourself and internally beat yourself up.*

Breeding the horses and selling the offspring has been another saving grace for me. Over the years, the foals produced on the farm have led me to remarkable people. Many who have come forward to buy the foals have become friends and remain in contact years later. Some connect with me in amazing ways and have often just appeared at the right moment throughout this journey. That is, sometimes by phone or message and sometimes in person. Incredibly, they seem to contact me at just some of the moments when I'm at my lowest and unfortunately not able to think of others, only myself. However, they are such generous people that they always have me in their thoughts. This all sounds a bit weird I know, and I don't know how their intuition tells them it's time to contact me, but it happens. Now that my road is less twisting and potholed I find I am tuning into them too. I owe them huge debts of gratitude for lifting me up and being there for me and I hope that I will live long enough to repay these special moments.

- *Whatever you focus on you will get more off. Focus your energies on friends and the way forwards and you will get it in abundance. Focus your incantations on yourself and build yourself up. If you're a woman who has given birth, it's like being in labour. It's a hard day's work and the reward at the end will be amazing. You will have a life and freedom. As the airlines say, 'Put your own oxygen mask on first before helping others'.*

The marks of success

Writing this book has helped remind me all that I have achieved. It was easy to become fixated on the failure of our marriage and carry the blame for it, and in doing so I forgot all the great things I accomplished. Now I have a written reminder of my successes and instead of guilt, I can feel the pride and joy of those achievements. Without my business plan and designs, we would not have been successful in getting the planning permission to build our own farm. Once we had that, I built a model for direct selling all our produce around the country and abroad. I loved the work and building business networks and making new online friends, many of whom I am still in touch with today. William constantly gave me a verbal bashing about being useless (I think that is known as gaslighting). Over a period, I began to doubt my ability to succeed at anything and took the blame for anything that went wrong. This has reminded me just how strong, resilient and successful I am and how many happy memories I have of the work I did. In future, I will use this experience to remind myself that I can achieve anything I put my mind and heart into.

- *Don't let your confidence in yourself be eroded by lies. Check very carefully that you are not adopting a belief as a truth. If you have a partner who is blaming you, maybe it is an indication that they are not the right person for you. Keep reminding yourself of your worthiness and that what you need is a partner who is there to respect and support you not apportion blame. I believe a solid relationship should be both partners sharing the load, whether for good or bad. Remember happy times as that and celebrate your success and achievements with yourself. Don't let a gas lighter steal those happy times.*

The house sale and removals

Summer 2017 and we got a firm offer for the house and part of the farm, Connor got his A levels and was accepted at university. I thought for a while I was nearly through the tunnel! I asked for the rest of the ground to be marketed immediately so that our finances could be sorted all at once. The agents were reluctant in case the house sale fell through and although I argued the case for delaying completion until after the house completion, if we got a sale, William wouldn't agree to sell the ground as he wanted to buy it. I was fine with this and insisted it was at full open market price. There was the difficulty. According to William's comments and letter, he clearly believed that I had had enough money already and should be giving him the land. (This was despite the Financial Order instructions, which William completely disregarded.) In the event, the agents wouldn't market the land until after the house sold, so it was a stalemate for a while. Reflecting on this leads me to think that William had a big say in when the ground was marketed and I have let the agents know that they have lacked equality in their treatment of the land sale. The completion was set for October and Connor took up his place at university in September. As there was going to be no need to provide a home for Connor, I decided to move out. The court had ordered that we agree to the split of furniture between us. I made a list of everything and asked William to decide what he wanted. He refused. I called in a removal man and William walked around the house with us as he listed items to remove. William objected to as much as possible, even a desk he had given to Connor and a little wardrobe and wood chest of little value but full of memories for Connor. Connor later asked his Dad if he could have the items and was told he couldn't have them anywhere where I would be. Even when he moved out of halls at university and into his student house, his father wouldn't lend him a plate and cup let alone any furniture. I had privately given the date to remove my furniture to the removal men and had arranged to store my share of the furniture at a friend's house. I had also decided not to leave the farm completely in case the sale fell through, and to move into one of the log cabins. Unfortunately, I lived in a very small community and confidentiality was totally lacking. Somehow, and my suspicion was the son of the remover, who was a friend of William's brother, the removal date became known to William. On the day, William went out early as he had a job to do for his brother, but not before he had bolted the bedroom door and put a notice on it threatening none to enter or remove any furniture. The furniture he referred to was my bed!

The removal men started moving other items and I phoned my solicitor to ask for help. As I was doing this, William arrived back. He went straight to the removers and threatened them that if they removed any items from the bedroom, they would not be leaving as he had parked the excavator across the drive. They were unnerved and started to unload what they had already loaded. I asked the solicitor to speak to William, but William was very angry and determined I wasn't going to have my bed. I went and reminded the removers that I had paid in advance and they were working for me and the bed was on the list to be moved. However, they only agreed to carry on if I left the items William had now decided he wanted and, in desperation, I agreed. I have learnt from Connor that William subsequently left the bed and mattress outside. When Connor went to ask his Dad for help with furniture and finance for his student house William showed him the destroyed bed, which he made sure the mice had well used.

This was once again a show of William's control, not just over me but also the removal men. I have since read that, particularly in rural communities, many people close ranks with the abuser and victims suffer further. I certainly felt that was true in my case.

- *If you find yourself in the same situation, try and get someone away from the area to do your removals. If you are in a small community, always try and get a solicitor and any other help and support from further afield. You are less likely to run up against people taking sides and making judgements! On the day of moving, get friends and family to help you.*

Removing myself

Once the furniture had departed I moved my clothes to the holiday let log cabin and for a few nights felt safer, like I had a place to myself. I had told Connor and friends where I was and took my security cameras with me. I went back to the house every day as the wi-fi I needed for work was there. For a couple of days, William didn't catch on that I was in the cabin, but when he did he left a basket of his dirty washing inside the back door of the cabin. The security camera didn't cover that door, so I couldn't prove anything but took the basket back unwashed and said nothing. The completion date was set, so I decided to take a week away. Before leaving I was at a friend's who was going to have Connor's dog while I was away. Suddenly, my phone alerted me to the fact that the security camera had been tripped in the cabin. Sure enough, it was William prowling around the cabin. I was frightened, and my friend's husband suggested calling the police and he would come back with me and wait for the police. We got to the top of the drive and waited for the police who arrived twenty minutes later. As we drove down the drive William was driving up. The police came in and checked the place for any signs of a break-in. One bedroom window had been forced. They made sure I was safe and said there was little they could do as it was really a civil matter! As William was co-owner of the farm and cabin, he had every right to enter. They suggested they would go to the house and have a word with him and suggest he didn't repeat his actions. Unsurprisingly, this didn't happen as William hadn't returned to the house. I expect he was parked behind a hedge waiting for the police to leave. They told me they would try telephoning him and later informed me this hadn't been a success either. I was so worried and stressed I decided to stay at the friend's for the night and go on my holiday from there. Throughout the week the camera recorded an almost daily visit from William to the cabin. He would put letters in front of the camera or make gestures. Another little control tweak. In the end, I didn't check the camera when I was notified as I wanted a week to myself.

This was stalking which I believe is considered a crime, but not seen as such by many, because William and I were once married. The police just looked at it from the wrong angle and called it a bit of a domestic! I believe there is great apathy when it comes to these situations between couples who have split up. At the time the laws regarding coercive control, abuse and stalking were all very new and maybe the training of professionals is now much better. I know better now and would keep calling the police and reminding them what this really is. I would advise anyone else to do the same. As I've already stated, I am now emotionally stronger, more resilient and in a much safer place mentally and physically. It is easier to be more objective.

- *If you're in the midst of a similar situation, just call the police and while you wait for them suck a lemon or douse yourself with cold water as it helps ground you. Make sure you impress on the police that this is an abuser and controller at work and you know it is criminal behaviour. If you believe they have difficulty because the person is a previous partner, ask them what they would do if it was a complete stranger.*

Mental health games

William had always been one for leaving notes of instructions on the table for me to find and after the financial remedy order and our official divorce in December 2016, they increased in frequency. They were about my 'mental illness' in the main and drifted onto topics such as my evil greedy nature. To ensure I got his message he wrote lengthy epistles to my stepdaughters, my friends and my solicitor. To the latter, he requested that under their duty of care to clients they should take action against me! While writing this and looking back on the raft of notes I still shake with emotion at the content and the bile and venom expressed. In my new home, I have a lemon tree and there are times when I need to suck on a few lemons to ground myself and remind myself that I am safe. William has a misguided notion of the 'without prejudice' term. He seems to believe he can use the term in his letters and write anything he likes about me to others, and whatever he likes to me, without it becoming an open document. This is not the case as the term only protects to a certain degree when in the court arena. Letters written to me are my property and therefore I feel can be published and shown to the world at large outside the courtroom.

- *Anyone on the receiving end of these kinds of malicious communications, please ground yourself before reading. If necessary get a friend to read them. Do not destroy them as they can be submitted to the police and the 'without prejudice' term has no meaning when it comes to disclosing this kind of evidence. Remember, this is domestic abuse evidence, which is a crime. Have some incantations ready for these times and go and smile and repeat them to yourself in front of the mirror. Love yourself and see all your strengths and know you are resilient and a survivor.*

As with most house sales, vacant possession was required, so the massive job of clearing and tidying the farm house and buildings started. Over the years, William had collected a variety of junk which needed moving, and there was silage plastic and rubbish, as well as a barn full of tools, freezers, lawn mowers, decorating equipment and the usual household detritus to be sorted out. William didn't believe that the financial remedy order section stating that we should divide this equally was applicable to him. He had a different set of rules and completely ignored the court. I was exhausted with the whole thing and so cleaned up and gave up trying to get half shares in the mowers and strimmers. William removed everything and I just let it go as I wanted it all to end and thought that this would be a more peaceful and quicker route. The end result was that William left all the rubbish and unwanted bits and made no attempt to clear it. I asked William what he planned to do about the remaining rubbish and items. He was unresponsive so I told him I would order a skip for the big rubbish items and then organise a friend's four-wheel drive to tow a trailer full of the remaining unsold and unwanted items to the local auction. I enlisted my daughters' help and a couple of friends. William was in the house and remained there all morning while we loaded up the items and cleaned up the barn. Although the barn was only yards from the back door of the house William did not make any attempt to come and help. When it was finally done, William ran out of the house and snatched the keys from the ignition of the vehicle, and demanded we unload the trailer as he wanted various items. I was gutted that he had watched us all morning and not said a word and then took this stance. At no time had he said he wanted any of it. After unloading a few of the things he said he wanted he returned the keys and so I could take the rest to the auction. Needless to say, everyone was a bit unnerved by his behaviour. I went the next morning with a friend and delivered the stuff to the auction yard. Later that day, I had a phone call from the auction house stating that they had had a visit from William demanding all items be withdrawn from the sale. In the event and after much discussion, they allowed William to remove two or three items and store them round the back for later collection. In return William allowed the rest to be entered into the sale. The items he removed were still round the back some three months later and to my knowledge could still be there. I believe William only did that to show the auction house who was the boss. As with so many other incidents, it seems that my instructions were overlooked and ignored. William could be very aggressive and assertive and as with so many of these incidents, he was from a well-known and influential family in the small rural pond. I was an incomer and often felt that people took William's view that I was the b...ch who stole everything off him! Everywhere he went, he told the story of me stealing his farm. As it is a very patriarchal community, I don't suppose anyone wondered what he was talking about. After all, a few years before it was just some fields. I expect they believe it was William who got the planning permission and built a business. How I wish I had had some lessons in assertiveness, but at the time all I wanted was to get away. Even now I get shivers when it comes to returning to the area for any reason. The more recent 'incomers' are fine, but many of the families who have been in the area for many years do not speak. Rural community justice in action!

- *Don't let public opinion deter you. It is very often distorted. It's like fake news! Don't try to convince them to change their opinions either. They are usually self-centred, small-minded people who have never left their local area. To boot, they have little education or knowledge of topics such as domestic abuse. They were probably abused themselves and have grown up with a distorted sense of right and wrong. Education will enlighten their children hopefully so that future generations will be more alert and prepared to rise up against such abuse.*

Completion, but only the house

Finally, the house completion date arrived. Typically, William had left the clearing up and cleaning to me and I was so keen to get the sale finished I did it. I got the window cleaners, the carpet cleaners, the skips for the rubbish. I organised the removal of the silage plastics and rubbish to recyclers and mending of fences so that all was in order for our buyers. It was a long slog. The few hiccups were caused by William's continuing non-acceptance that this was real. He refused to accept that someone else was going to be the owner of our house and continually ranted at me and anyone else who was nearby, about how I had stolen everything off him. Unfortunately, in a few instances, I believe this mud stuck and the local community became a place where I felt very mixed emotions. Some clearly didn't get involved in having a view on something they knew nothing about. Others, for their own reasons, seemed to me to take our divorce on a personal level. Of course, there were also those admirable supporters of me who made my life much more bearable during this period. I was overjoyed at last being free, well nearly, and starting again. I now reflect that this was not the end. It was nearer the beginning of the journey of rebuilding myself and overcoming low self-esteem and confidence. It was coupled with a giant amount of guilt, grief and regrets. All of these emotions were a bit unexpected and followed very closely on the back of the relief of finally being able to move away from William. However, our physical distance was nowhere near enough miles apart to give me peace. I now realise this was not the end at all, it was the beginning of a side of William that I hadn't really met before. For me too, the self-doubt, terrors, nightmares and fear started and of course the voices, convincing me of my faults and that I was as useless as William had stated. Regaining myself was going to be more of a challenge than the last twenty-five years at times. William's personality was that of a chameleon and I suppose, when a coercive controller believes themselves to be wronged, they change up a gear in their venomous actions and behaviours. I was out and free..... but only briefly. It is an appropriate time for me to stop this book and rest and recover my strength and ground myself before writing on. Post-traumatic stress disorder, to my mind, is being revisited by trauma. I have to reframe the experiences before I can start the next chapter.

- *Never, never, never allow yourself to be talked into stage payments and delay in divorce and finances. Make sure there is a single decisive cut. Do not feel sorry for or guilty because you are the partner who wants the divorce. In many potential narcissist divorce cases, it is the empath who petitions. It doesn't make you wrong or justify lesser settlements. Do not allow anyone to talk you out of getting your own oxygen mask on and helping yourself. Until you are on an even keel, you can't help your children, family or friends. So concentrate on your own needs first.*

Finding a safe place to live

Reading what I have written, I believe many may think that I chose to move to Spain because I wanted a life in the sun, or because I had met someone else and fancied a jolly or indeed that I did so fantastically well financially, I could afford it. In many ways, the reverse is true. Fear and finances made the decision for the move to Spain. I was afraid of the monster William seemed to have become. I was afraid that he would never be reasonable or move on with his life. The endless notes and letters which appeared in the dark of the night gave me the jitters. As I had accepted a very low settlement in exchange for my freedom, I was not able to afford the high-priced property in the UK. I didn't feel like I belonged anywhere as I had been isolated on the farm for so many years. A friend suggested Spain, as she had lived there for a good number of years. She explained that there were very reasonable places to buy or rent and that the overall cost of living was much cheaper. I decided to investigate whether I could move to Spain or another country and still be able to see my family and friends as well as get work. Now that I am in a safer and more emotionally stable place, I do find that some of the horror and fear is dissipating. It is only when a memory pops back in that I remember how severe the daily anxiety was.

After moving out of the farm, the barrage of letters, texts and emails increased over time with every step I took away from William. Wherever I was living in the UK, he somehow found me and there would be envelopes left on my car windscreen or dropped through the letterbox. It always made me anxious that he had been somewhere nearby stalking me. It was wearying and frightening, especially when I was alone at night. It was his way of trying to regain and exert control, and I found it seriously worrying. Several friends, who I stayed with at times, were also unnerved by it.

The stalking continued wherever I went. Somehow, he knew when I was away from the area for work and where I was. I carefully checked my social media friends and contacts and over time withdrew from engaging with most of it. I kept my messages and movements and photos to a small circle of close friends and family. This worked but had the effect of making me feel I had lost my freedom and was always looking over my shoulder. The arguments over the divorce and the reaction of his family had started me thinking that I needed to be much further away in order to feel safe and that I wasn't being constantly watched.

I considered the Midlands where I had grown up, but hadn't got any connections left in the area. Then I thought about gravitating towards London, after all a big city is easier to get lost in. This didn't sit well, because although I enjoy going to work in the city, I have always lived a more rural life. The thought of managing to keep my dog in

London wasn't my idea of regaining peace in my life. I went to Scotland to see how I felt about being there but it didn't seem far enough, I felt a bit exposed for some reason even though William had no connections there. I went to the USA to see if I could settle near my family out there but didn't feel safe there either. The part of the country where my family lives is very spread out so the 'being near' them would actually have meant at least half an hour's drive. At the same time, I didn't want my family and friends to have to be anxious and worried and looking after me. I wanted to be free and independent and safe from William. Well, in fact, at the stage where I didn't ever have to consider him!

After investigating all these, I started thinking of what my friend had said about Spain. It matched many of my needs. I had been to Spain with my first husband and the girls and we'd had the most wonderful holidays. I had also visited my friend on the Costa del Sol and Connor and I had really enjoyed feeling like we had a second home with her. This gave me warm and happy feelings when I thought about it, which in turn made me feel safer.

I arranged to fly out and although I kept very quiet about my plans, somehow William found out and he stalked me through social media messages. I spent the first day of my house-hunting visit blocking everyone from all my social media so I could relax and travel around looking to see if any of it felt like home. Inside I was very upset and beating myself up for running away. I looked at the landscape and wondered how would I get used to the dry land and sea instead of the lush green fields and woodland I had always known. I decided that if I could find a place in the country similar to where I had been living, it would be a small enough step for me to manage. I first went back to where I had stayed with my friend, but there was nothing that attracted me to live there. In the ten years since I had visited, there had been an explosion of apartments and bars, and it was all too much of a tourist hub for me to find peace.

I was fortunate that the man who was finding property for me suggested looking up the coast in an area I had never been. I drove up there and found that I felt a connection with the more rural area and its avocado and mango groves. I felt peaceful and calm and not so many miles from home and Connor, my family and friends.

That is how I came to be where I am today. Fear brought me here and now I'm glad it did. I can now look at the move as an adventure. However, in the first few days and months, it was quite terrifying. For many years, I hadn't been independent and made any of my own choices and now here I was in a strange country and couldn't speak any Spanish! Friends helped me move out here and I was in a meltdown once they left. I am crying now as I write and I remember the terrible fear that was gripping me. In my head were William's words about how I was a useless person who couldn't make it on my own and how unsuccessful I was at everything in life.

I was alone amongst neighbours who didn't speak English and only Connor and the two friends who helped me move there knew where I was. Some nights were completely sleepless because of my constant worry that William and his stalkers would find me. I use the word stalker now, but at the time I really didn't realise this was what it was. I was so moulded into thinking the divorce and everything was my fault and therefore the blaming and scathing poisonous letters and messages were my own fault.

It has taken many, many hours of counselling to straighten my thinking and I still beat myself up regularly, despite the therapy.

The universe works in an amazing way and I feel it has somehow brought me to a place where I am safe and have made many new friends of all nationalities, as well as preserved the friendships back in the UK. In a way, the coronavirus pandemic has strengthened all my relationships as we have all had to turn to the digital world and video calls to keep ourselves going.

It greatly increased the speed at which I learnt Spanish and I can now engage in simple conversations, especially with my neighbours. Although my competence at the language doesn't yet allow me to talk about my fears and the past, (and in a way I don't want to), I now feel like I belong here and this is my home. I feel safer and not so worried about anyone knowing my location. Although I do have times when I lack confidence, they are much less severe and devastating to my well-being than when I first arrived.

I can't explain to my neighbours and friends here, but I think that if I was ever feeling unsafe or if William found me and threatened me, they would come to my rescue. I no longer feel that I ran and hid from William. Nowadays I choose to believe I did it to start my new adventure. If I were ever to repeat this, I would most definitely do it differently. For some reason, I didn't equate William's behaviour as stalking neither did the police at that time, and in my desire to get away I let it go. I am now stronger and more confident and would not let this go.

- *If you are faced with similar situations, keep going. Get a friend to help press your case if you need support. If you feel you are not being listened to by your local police, refer matters to a higher ranking department. Don't be intimidated and frightened to let anyone know where you are, because of the threat of repercussions from an ex-partner.*

After Life

Writing this first part of my story left me completely exhausted mentally and emotionally. I have taken a bit of time and changed my method in order to fortify myself enough to write the next chapters. I have been researching what sort of self-help and development I need to do to let go of the mixed emotions of the past and move forward. Self-awareness is one of the foundations of success, so I am working on my thoughts and feelings and the way in which I formulate my friendships and relationships. Alongside my book of life after the sale of the farmhouse, I am writing my reflections now that there is a bit more time and distance between me and the past. At the moment, we are in the middle of the global coronavirus crisis and so I have many days totally alone. It has its benefits as I am in a safe place to reflect on my past and how I want to use that to shape my future. I am now feeling strong enough to go back in time and look at what happened next.

I was so relieved when we finally completed the house sale and I could move out. In my naive mind, I thought it was nearly the end. Reflecting on that now it is more like the beginning of the next chapter. With regards to the abusive behaviour, it got much worse.

It didn't take William very long to track down my new address, (I had moved to a friend's bungalow about five miles away.) Very soon the malicious notes started arriving. They would greet me when I got in my car in the mornings, stuck under the windscreen wipers. Or hand-delivered in the letterbox. Unbelievably, I didn't think of this as stalking and just put up with it. I rang my solicitor a few times to ask for advice.

Reflecting on this I would now always call the police and press my point. At the time I was still holding the limiting belief that I had brought this on myself by leaving William and the marriage. I have done a lot of self-blame for a large number of years and nowadays I have stopped beating myself up (nearly!) or blaming. At the time, I remember thinking of calling the police, but my previous experience over the rape had not met with the best response, and I didn't feel strong enough to go through the humiliation again.

- *If you are in a similar situation, make sure you do report all these events, no matter how trivial. If you have asked your ex-partner to stop contacting and they continue to harass you, go for a no-contact order. All the little previous instances which are recorded will be evidence for you. Even if you have to have a contact for the sake of children, putting in strong boundaries will help.*

After the sale of the farmhouse, we still had the remaining farmland to sell. Against my better judgement and wishes, the agents had advised us not to market the land until the house sale was completed. The impact of this was a delay and overall prolonged sale, something I really wasn't happy with. However, I agreed and reluctantly went along with their advice. Immediately after the house sale had completed, I asked the agents to start marketing the ground. That was when more problems started. It became clear that William had been talking to the agents and wanted to keep the remaining ground for himself. Initially, William did not want to give me any money for the ground but was then persuaded by the agents to make an offer. William made a minimal offer as he really felt, in his words, that he had bought the ground twice and I had done nothing over the twenty years to contribute to the increased value of the farm. This was despite the very clear apportionment and instructions of assets in the financial remedy order. I now realise that in an abuser's world there is only their version of the truth and so whatever the court had indicated bore no resemblance to what was William's world. He did not believe I deserved a share in the assets, so why should he buy me out at open market value? Added to this was the fact that the agents required a new set of terms and conditions signing in order to market the remaining acres of grounds. As you might expect, William would not sign the terms and conditions and this eventually led, after several months of waiting, to another court application to direct William to sign and put the land on the market. Anxiety and stress had now returned to my life. I had been excited when we sold the house to think that my relationship with William was nearly at an end. I had started my new business and had a plan for its development once I received my share of the sale proceeds. Now William was becoming very difficult to communicate with and every little thing to do with the old farm businesses and the sale of the ground was largely aggressive, argumentative and very stressful. Five months after the sale of the house, we went to court and had an order to market the ground with two agents at full market value.

Two months later, and with two agents instructed, we arranged a meeting to walk the ground and discuss the values and marketing strategy. I arrived for the meeting as did both agents. However, William chose to stay away. He had informed one of the agents of this intention and unfortunately, that agent did not manage to encourage him to come along. I knew it was a bad idea to continue with the meeting with just the three of us, but the agents assured me it would be okay. It was not okay. William's reaction to the valuation report and marketing strategy was to say that it was inaccurate and that the agents had acted for me not him. Inevitably, this resulted in another application to the court to get William to the communication table and compel him to purchase the ground at the full open market value. This kind of delay became a part of everyday life for me and was so wearing. The fact that the agents seemed to have fallen prey to William's behaviours was also very disconcerting. Couple this with a sort of institutionalised sexist inequality, where whatever the man says carries more weight and I found the whole situation like one of pushing water up a steep mountain. The emotional impact and stress were huge and I can fully understand why many people give up their fight for equality in preference for some good quality mental health.

- *This is very much the tactics of delay and continuing control. Beware of the effect and costs of such delays. You need to keep reporting criminal behaviours to the police and let your legal adviser know as well. If necessary, find national support organisations and contact them.*

What was left

When William became aware that in all likelihood he was going to have to pay the full market price for the remaining land, a number of issues arose. The main one was that suddenly he remembered various debts that I allegedly owed him. Mysteriously although it had taken us two years to get a financial remedy order agreed, he had forgotten these debts at the time of the order in 2016. So the next application to the court for marketing the ground was hijacked by William presenting a lengthy and completely fraudulent document full of debts, misdemeanours, hearsay and reasons why he shouldn't pay me the full market value for the ground.

That year there was an extremely warm and dry spring and because William had not attended the initial walk round the ground he disagreed with both agents' ideas on marketing and kept asserting that the water supply was not good. It was a spring-fed supply and had never ever dried up, even though we had had dry periods before. Funnily enough, this year, the water suddenly dried up. This happened to be in the fields that I was using for my horses. I asked a friend to come and dig a couple of sumps in the ground which then promptly filled up with water. The gates to the field mysteriously opened and my livery horses got out and were loose on the road. In order to protect this, I put chains and padlocks around all of the gates along with wildlife cameras so that I could be sure that the horses remained safe.

A second walk of the ground was arranged with the agents and this time William was compelled to be present. Once again, overnight, the water had all dried up. In William's view, this devalued the ground. In the agent's view, as they had seen it with the water running, they didn't believe it presented a problem with their valuation. Indeed, I could show them video footage of the water flowing from the spring and the water holes full the night before. Interestingly, a neighbour who shared the spring supply rang in the afternoon of the walk to complain that his water supply had also dried up. William went up to see him and immediately located the source of the problem with the spring and was able to restore the water flow. Unfortunately, my wildlife cameras were not in the right position to capture what exactly was blocking the water supply.

In all honesty, I was still trying to make things right at this stage and feeling guilty for having failed to make the marriage work. Everything I did was because of that guilt so I still did not see the degree to which I was being manipulated, although I felt its constant pressure. I am now able to reframe these thoughts to some extent and treat myself with more respect. This has been an extraordinarily lengthy divorce and now I am managing my emotions better. I can now recognise when I am falling back into old Trish who is trying to be good enough and stop and adjust my thoughts. It has cost me dearly in terms of emotional impact and the finances of a therapist! However, there is no more worthy cause. I have advocated Connor to use the help of a counsellor if and when he needs and I hope to set him an example of how to be your best self and that it is no weakness to get help. It is a weakness to keep thinking you can solve everything alone.

- *Don't fall into the same trap. You are not guilty of anything. You are a victim of a manipulative abuser. Get professional help to come to terms with the what and why and move forward. Alone it is easy to fall back into the arms of the abuser, who of course you still have feelings for, even if it is resentment and hate. Learn how to deal with all the manipulative behaviour and help yourself recognise it in the future.*

More delay and the effect on me

Both land agents tried to encourage William to make a sensible offer to buy me out of the remaining land as this would not require the need to put it on the open market and would save on their fees. William refused, he wanted the ground for nothing, as he believed he was the one who had paid for it originally. He also felt that divorce had cost him enough already and that I wasn't worthy of anymore. He held to his belief that it was all his land and money. So there was no other option but to put the land on the open market, with him approved as priority purchaser if we had any offers. This would enable William to match the highest bid.

By the time we got to this point, I was getting very anxious about the degree of control William still exerted over my life. Symptoms of PTSD were starting to surface every time I had to meet him or communicate with him. I was still at the point where I believed what he had told me for years, that I was not worth it. I had also been taken by surprise at the lengths to which he went to cut off the water supply, loose animals out of the fields and generally do anything to sabotage the sale of the ground. None of this could be proven of course, but I knew it was him and that he was doing it to reduce the saleability of the ground. With hindsight, I believe I should have gone to the police. Even though it would have been difficult to prove that it was William's handiwork, at least they would have been obliged to take some notice if I had kept reporting these instances. At that time, I still lacked the confidence in myself to keep pressing the police. As they had virtually dismissed my rape allegation and the stalking, both as civil matters, I had little confidence that any of my other complaints would be heard and dealt with appropriately. I sincerely hope that I will never get myself into this kind of situation again. One of the great learnings while writing this book and reflecting is that I now see with a better perspective. Although I keep saying I have learnt a lot, I don't think that these kinds of pressures should be put on those who have suffered this kind of abuse. Why am I asked what I learnt from the situation as if it were some kind of college course I had been through? Actually, it was victimisation and I was the target of something horrifically abusive. The only thing I need to learn is that it wasn't my fault.

- *Do not try to forget these events as that will not help for the future or for your mental health. Start trying to look from an unemotional perspective and find the learnings. These will help you recognise any similar people in the future. Add your voice to some of the groups who campaign for better training and understanding from the police and legal professionals. This will help shed a light on these many covert behaviours and for those that follow. Understand that the reality is that it wasn't you. You were the target and not the cause. Get help from a professional to overcome the symptoms of what is now known as complex post-traumatic stress disorder.*

Connor's Education

Problems were also starting to arise from William's lack of engagement with Connor's education and he certainly didn't want to engage over any contributions towards his finances or the provision of a car or anything else for that matter. Despite the fact that Connor was still in full-time education, William would regularly declare that Connor was an adult and independent. If Connor asked his Dad for any kind of assistance, it would be rejected while at the same time William would tell Connor that I had stolen everything off him so I could pay.

For years I thought I was protecting Connor by leaving him out of the information loop. After several of his Dad's attacks, I realised that Connor was unwittingly being dragged into the middle, because he wasn't sure of the truth and whether his mother needed defending. I sat down and wrote a timeline of everything which had happened and every asset we had acquired and who had funded it, throughout our life together. Hopefully, I gave Connor an unbiased statement of facts. I told him this was not to fight his Dad with but merely for information so he knew the truth. I wanted Connor to be with me because we love and respect each other, and not because he felt I needed protection. I have since updated these facts twice so that William can never again put Connor into the middle of our divorce. I would recommend to anyone to do this much sooner than I did. It seems to have helped Connor to make his own way with his Dad and maintain a relationship on Connor's terms not controlled by his Dad.

- *Give your children as much age-appropriate information as possible. Make sure you give information in a dispassionate and unbiased way, such as a list. Often a third party who is not Mum or Dad can help children to be heard and hear their thoughts. Never let the child think or believe it is because of them. Help them to understand that they can still love both parents and won't be punished for that.*

Will life ever be normal?

Having surrendered my guns and licence after reporting William for attempted rape, and although I no longer have a use or need for a gun, I am still pushing for their return. This is mainly because I want to be the one who has the choice over when I sell my gun and to whom. It may be a bit pedantic, but it will be one more action that symbolises I have made my own decision and not had it made for me by William, the police or anyone else. Problems still exist in getting back mine and Connor's licences. Connor held a licence although he shared my guns. The police very properly enquired with my doctor for a report on my health and mental health. These came back positive and I was due to get my guns returned to me and Connor would also be allowed his licence, except that they had to get a report from William. Of course, I now realise that William was never going to release any part of the control he had exerted over me for so many years. The police asking him about me gave him the opportunity to say he believed that if my guns were returned to me I would pursue him and possibly shoot him. Despite everything I had said, my references had said and the doctor's report, this was all ignored because of William's words. The police informed me that I would be unable to have my guns returned until all of our finances were settled. As we still had the ground to sell, there was no possibility of this happening any time soon. (By way of an update, three years on because the funds for the sale of the ground are still in the court arena and in dispute, I am still unable to have my guns returned. Although the police have indicated that as soon as Connor has got a place of his own he will be allowed to have his licences and keep a gun.)

The problem with securing the return of my guns was not limited to the attitude of the police force and seems to be throughout all the systems. In my case, the legal system and the government have also been stumbling blocks. I do not think that this discrimination is intentional, it is merely the way the systems are set up. However, as with many policies, they need to be urgently reviewed. This should be to ensure that all forms of abuse and potential for abuse are safeguarded against. I have found that throughout the whole divorce process and everyone I have come into contact with, the potential William has had to continue his coercive controlling behaviour has been supported by many of these systems and policies. It is tempting to leave it all and never try to claim my guns or complain about the systems. However, there is something in me that wants to set an example to Connor, and which says do not put up and shut up, make a noise and make a change happen. If no one complains, all these abuses by society and inequalities can continue. Having felt the stress of it all, I believe I want to do my best to help make it better for future generations and make the change happen.

> • *The existing systems are sometimes very much in need of reform and modernising. Do what you can to help bring that about. Make complaints about the inefficiency and failings of a system wherever you find it. You will practice your assertiveness in the process and become a part of a new future. If you say nothing and just accept things, there will always be inequalities. It is the service users who enlighten the policy-makers. Be a part of new policy-making whenever you can.*

Family sticks together

I believe William's family was also enlisted to continue threats and bullying in a variety of ways. One action was over a loan that I had had with William's mother, Linda, a number of years before. The loan was towards a property. This had been a private verbal agreement and I had always paid Linda a substantial amount of interest each year. She had initially requested that I match the interest she would have had, had the money remained in her building society. As the interest rates had sunk to ridiculously low levels, I made up the amount of interest because I felt that was fairer. As part of the divorce settlement, William was pushing for me to sell the property. This meant that until the sale was complete there were no students or rent coming in. I therefore agreed with Linda to reduce the interest to a minimum and make a single payment from the proceeds of the sale. Unfortunately, the sale took a long time, and in the interim Linda had a stroke and William's elder sister and his brother were appointed attorneys. Shortly after the sale had completed and I repaid the loan and interest, I started receiving threatening letters from his brother and sister. The letters were making demands for unpaid interest. Although there was no formal loan agreement, they had calculated the interest based on rates that I had previously paid Linda while students were paying rent. Many of these letters were accompanied by William's threatening words. It took several months before my explanations as to what interest was due and that it had all been paid were accepted. It is now three years ago and I have not received any summons to court for the unofficial interest. I believe they have possibly reduced their claim.

I now recognise that all my loans and liabilities should have been listed in full in the financial remedy order and that they should have been shared equally with William. After the sale of the property, he took half of the proceeds of the sale but had never shared half of the costs. I lost £..000 on the sale of the student house and also had to pay William £.000. This was a total loss to me of £..000. The financial remedy order should have been drawn up to include this. It is just another example of how keen I was to get out of our marriage, so I shouldered all the burden of debts. At the time, I also thought that William would be as reasonable and fair as me in the divorce. After all, I was the 'guilty' party wanting out of the marriage but didn't believe William to be the monster he has now shown himself to be.

- *It is very difficult at a time of the financial settlement to put aside your feelings and just concentrate on the facts. Get a friend to help you look objectively at your settlement and at the wording to ensure it makes sense to them. Because you know your story, your brain fills in gaps for you at times, which a friend's brain won't. For all financial settlements, you need an objective view not an emotional one. Don't forget that an abuser will know how to trigger the empath in you. Get someone independent to scrutinise your agreement as they don't have the same emotions. Don't worry about what is best for your ex-partner financially. Instead, think about what is best for you and your future.*

Now is not the time for reflection

I have jumped forward to record the latest attempt at undermining and controlling me. Instead of looking back, I'm in it at the moment.

A few days ago, William requested the tax returns for the two farm businesses that we are still in partnership together. This has happened because all court dates since April 2019 have been adjourned, so there is still no resolution for me as to when the partnerships can be dissolved and I can be properly free of him. Of course, William isn't at all concerned because this way he can maintain his influence over my life. I forwarded the tax returns and yesterday had an email from MY solicitor, who informed me that William and his accountants have contacted him directly for permission to discuss the sale of the farm and land. I am mystified, as was my solicitor. We cannot understand why William would think that I would instruct and pay my solicitor to liaise with him and his accountants. I suspect this is yet another of William's little schemes to get me to pay for his life.

Oh dear! he's really trying to turn the screws. My solicitor received a letter from his solicitor asking for the accountants to contact my solicitor. What's he on? I'm not about to let my solicitor collaborate with William!

Also, he has made accusations of libellous activity because I posted some information on social media when I made a fund-raising page in an effort to get some financial support to pay towards my legal bills. He's picked up on that and is trying to get my solicitor to tell me to remove it. Actually, my solicitor isn't my keeper, and nothing is libellous as I don't name William and I'm telling the truth.

On re-reading this, I can see a note of rising panic in my writing and yet again I am trying to make all things right. Something reached the maximum in me just after I wrote this in January 2020, and I stopped being endlessly obliging and trying to settle the matter. Now I have stopped all communication and await a final court hearing. Owing to the delays and changes William keeps making to his claim against me, the length of the hearing is now three days! This and Coronavirus meant that it is unlikely to be listed before 2021. Now that I have resolved to present my case to the court, I feel more relaxed and peaceful. I am not sure if putting my faith in a judge to hold William to account is the right decision, but only time will tell.

- *You may find it very hard to do but no contact or low contact is the best way forward with this. Do not keep those texts and messages which confuse your emotions into thinking your abuser loves you despite all their behaviour. Recognise that this is just the cycle of destruction and if you jump back in, you will go round again. Email or message your solicitor very regularly to get a court date fixed. Ring and message and petition the court daily. Let them know what dire straits you are in. This gives you a feeling of taking action rather than reacting to the abuser all the time.*

The next development is that the government agency has now started reclaiming our inactivated entitlements. The farm businesses gained entitlements which we still hold jointly, and they match our acreage of land. They enable us to make an annual claim for financial support providing we observe environmental and animal welfare rules. As we sold one of the farms in 2017 and some more land the next year, our acreage has reduced and therefore we are unable to use all our entitlements. We have two years to sell or lease the inactivated entitlements or lose them to the national reserve. Originally, William was going to purchase the ground and therefore asked the court to order that he be able to buy the entitlements. As this didn't happen, he lost this status and has steadfastly refused to consent to either of these solutions and we have now lost our first lot of entitlements. While this is not a huge sum of money, it is yet another instance of William controlling my finances and his decisions carrying more weight than mine. Without his consent to sell or lease these, I am stuck with waiting for them to be reclaimed. I have this in part of my argument for court and I am claiming the full value for half of the entitlements.

While the case keeps getting adjourned, it is now becoming a matter of urgency that this is dealt with or we both lose out. Originally, I thought the possibility of losing money would motivate William to progress our settlement as quickly as possible. It has become very apparent that by far the bigger motivation for him is to pursue me and control me to the very last moment. I am not sure that even if a court tells him it is final, he will accept the situation. Once again, at the very last minute, William consented to the sale of our inactivated entitlements. However, the transfer has taken a very long time and I still await the payment for them. Recent communications with the agency indicate that they have once again listened to William's version of events and I am now ignored by them when I ask for information. More water up the mountain! As this is a matter between the business partnerships and the agency, my solicitor cannot get involved. However, I am just compiling a report and complaint to send to my MP regarding the injustice of their actions.

- *Believe in yourself and the truths you are telling. The truth may be refuted by the abuser for a while, but eventually has to be admitted when you present evidence. Don't be misled into thinking that the unreal truth from the abuser will win the day. They tend to often change their version of the truth, which will support your truth and evidence the discrepancy. Be patient and try not to worry. It's like slowly, slowly, catch the monkey.*

First realisation of narcissism

I read an interesting article about divorcing a narcissist on *Psychology Today*. I think it's the first time I've really understood that William is potentially an extreme narcissist. Every word of the article is a real indication of who he is and could be written specifically about him. Interestingly, a friend I told about this suggested I reframe the way I think about my experiences. She suggested that actually William had helped me find a muscle I didn't know I had, in terms of resilience and growth.

Overnight, I thought about a number of ways I could start flexing and toning that muscle.

One way I could do it is to write a series of articles for others to enable them to spot the abuser in their relationship a lot earlier than I did. Maybe I can even develop that muscle into providing coaching and self-rehabilitation courses for those who want help surviving or recovering their self-esteem after the trauma. Finally, call me slow, but I am only just fully understanding what has been happening. At last, I can feel the freedom from blaming myself for everything that went wrong between us and is inevitably going wrong with the divorce process. This is not my making, this is the world of an abuser and potential narcissist, whose reality changes to suit his needs on a regular basis. Unfortunately, none of it has a basis in reality, honesty, fairness and truth. Now I really feel empowered.

- *Flex and tone your muscles. It may have been a few years so take it gently. Your muscle memory will click-in though and help you forward. Write it all down. Start with just bullet points and what you first think of. Then go over each point and write all you remember. Like me, you may want to publish your thoughts in the hope it helps others to not feel alone. Or you may want to burn them ceremoniously one day to rid yourself of that past.*

Delay and destroy

William's trail of delay. I have written this down to remind myself of what William has managed to delay so far. None of these delays could possibly have been in his best interests and can only have been to frustrate and control me.

Subsequent to our divorce and financial remedy order of November 2016, we were obliged to put our farm on the market and sell it. This was done in two parts. We found a buyer for the farmhouse and a few acres and had an offer the following June. Completion of the sale was in October of that same year. I pushed for the marketing of the remaining ground from the time of the June offer, so that potentially both the sales could have been completed at the same time. William had been keen to retain the remaining ground. I had no concerns about this but wanted him to buy it at open market value. William did not believe that he should have to pay that value or anything at all. He believed I had stolen enough!

Two years after the financial remedy order, I went back to court to get William to sign the instructions for the sale of the remaining land. The judge ordered that this must happen. At the same time, William requested he be the preferred buyer and alleged that I owed him money. In the order in June that year the judge instructed that the land be sold on the open market and that William could be the preferred purchaser by matching the highest open market offer and completing within 14 days of the matched offer. The judge further instructed that all outstanding monies owed to the parties be settled at the time of completion of this sale. The judge asked for William's list of what he alleged was owed but William hadn't got one. The judge ordered that he had to furnish the list within two weeks and I would also be given two weeks to respond.

William's further tactic was to act in person as he had seemingly disinstructed his solicitor after the sale of the farm the previous year.

After the court order in July, William had furnished his list as described above which consisted of many thousands of pounds that he apparently believed I owed him. I responded and clarified that he had in fact been paid in full for all the expenses which were real (but not for any that were made up). I sent extensive notes and evidence of my bills which had been set against some of the costs he claimed. There were several claims which I did not believe were correct. One such instance was an alleged purchase of sheep from William's mother before our divorce and the financial remedy order. I was never aware of this transaction and certainly, no sheep from his mother ever appeared at our farm. When questioned, William claimed that the sheep had been stolen, which was why I was unaware of them and that it was my responsibility as I should have put an insurance claim in for them! There was also a bill from William's sister's company for work done one month before we divorced. Even though this was supposed to have taken place less than four weeks before the financial remedy order and was work for our farm partnership, I was unaware of it and William informed the court that he had 'forgotten' it in the original farm sale completion. These additional farm costs which he was trying to claim of me had also not been included in our farm accounts submitted to HMRC. This totalled £...000 maximum.

I was somewhat taken aback by the fact that William could make allegations which were not evidenced or substantiated in any way, and it was down to me to prove I was innocent. I believed our legal system to operate the other way round, but no one ever asked William to provide evidence. As I now know, this was a licence for the abuser in my life to allege whatever he believed to be the truth in his world, regardless of the reality.

- *Be prepared. A narcissist's and an abuser's version of the truth can be very changeable on a daily basis and is their truth, not the actual truth. They are very capable of staging with certainty their fake truth in court after taking an oath. Be warned and make sure you have firm evidence of the actual truth. Sometimes our court system has to see the true colours of the abuser before it can take action.*

Payments and finances

Part of a farming income comes from what are known as single farm payments. This is the money received from the government based on animal welfare and maintaining certain farming practices. William had asked for a breakdown of the single farm payments and I had sent an extensive explanation of how they were broken down. There were also expenses set against this. I detailed everything from the Financial Order onwards, even though William had full possession of all of this information at the time the payments were made.

The remaining land was on the market and the final date for offers was August 2018. The offers were made in the form of a sealed bid and both William and I were required to be present at the agent's office when the received bids were opened. The day arrived and William did not attend the meeting and chose to be on the telephone instead, even though this was not the agreed procedure. In the event that no offers would be received, I had put in my own offer to ensure that William was not the only bidder at a ridiculously low price. My offer was proposed by the agents as the best offer. Despite William having been granted preferred purchaser status in June that year, he asked for twenty-four hours to consider the offer. It was also stipulated by the court that if William was the preferred bidder, he would be required to complete the purchase within fourteen days. One hour later, a late offer was entered by William's uncle which was then recommended as the best offer by the selling agents.

Are you totally exhausted with all this yet? If so, feel free to skip on a few pages. I am trying to convey the feeling of desperation caused by wading through treacle. I am hoping that those of you in a similar setting may use my experience to act differently and end the desperate situation sooner than I did. I have included all these details to try and give you an idea of how it feels to deal with the constant twists and turns in William's version of the truth and how that translated into an enormous delay. Seemingly, the whole manipulation thing pervaded all those who had anything to do with our case, and that included solicitors, judges, estate agents. His power to put the brakes on any progress and continue controlling me seemed endless at times. I was totally exhausted and anxious, thinking that my life would never improve. However, unlike you, I couldn't skip a few pages or court hearings.

End of August 2018, William decided not to match his uncle's offer, and therefore the planned completion date had William purchased it, would be delayed. This had the effect of putting the control back into the hands of William's family with them determining if and when I would get my share of the money.

November 2018 was the time set for William's uncle to complete the land purchase. A week before, yet again, William refused to sign the sales contract as he returned to the notion that 'I still owed him money'. On recommendation from the conveyancing solicitor, in order to get William to sign the sales contract and allow the sale to complete, I agreed to all proceeds of the sale being held by the solicitor until the 'money owing' issue was resolved. Urgent requests were sent to William to clarify what he felt was still owing.

In February, the next year, William had still not responded or supplied details, and so I made a further court application to get the money released.

Mid-April that year was the date for court. By the time this arrived, William had concocted a completely new list of debts and loans allegedly owed to his mother. Unfortunately, owing to a stroke, (which William blamed me for) his Mum had been frail for a year or more and had died the previous November. Thus William was now attempting to infer that I owed his mother's estate in his claim against me. His 'new' debts list totalled a staggering amount of nearly £60,000.

A week before the court, he had re-instructed his solicitor. Despite me making several offers before we went into the courtroom, William refused them all. In court, the judge ordered on the day that all supposed debts in connection with his mother's estate be removed from his list. If William wished to pursue these it would need to be done as a separate claim. He never did. The judge also urged both parties to offset as much as possible to reduce costs and court time. William's solicitor requested an adjournment, creating yet another delay, as he claimed he had only just been re-instructed even though he had been fully involved up to February, only two months before. The judge agreed and requested a final list from both William and me. She ordered a court hearing of four hours in order to consider what was left on the list and said she hoped we would be able to make an agreement before that date to save the costs.

A month later, statements were prepared and sent to the court regarding the final list. Once again, William's list had changed. Not only had he taken out the debts relating to his mother's estate, he had 'remembered' some new debts and was also now claiming all of the single farm payments, which was not what had been agreed in the financial remedy order. This was a completely new item and another attempt to create delay.

By June, the court had been sent and acknowledged receipt of all the paperwork but unfortunately had failed to forward it on to the judge. Because of the 'new item' regarding William's claim for the single farm payment, and the fact that the paperwork had not been received, the judge did not want to hear the case, when, yet again, we returned to court in late June.

William had instructed a very aggressive barrister for the day, who introduced another delay over the question of the dissolution of our farm partnerships. This date couldn't be arranged as the finances and final accounts could not be completed until the final list of costs was sorted out. The judge ordered that we do further questionnaires and responses and final draft accounts by August 2019 with a new court date to be set for after September. My solicitor was to type up the order and send it to the judge to perfect as soon as possible.

In August, all questionnaires and responses and accounts were done and a copy was sent to the court. My solicitor had also done the draft order for the June court hearing and chased up the court and the judge in July and August for approval of the order. We finally received a court date in early November.

In November, we arrived at court to find that the judge had finally received the missing paperwork from May, but had not received the draft order for the June hearing. As seemed to have become the norm, I made offers to settle outside the court and William rejected them. The judge dictated the order for the June hearing, all of which had been completed and then requested a final hearing be listed after January the following year. However, he thought from the issues now raised that this should be allocated two days in court and further half-day reading. As with every court appearance, the judge comments on the costs and the fact that all the money is being eaten up in court and legal costs.

I have been pragmatic and inadvertently played this game too long. The above timeline has served to remind me that it is William, not me, who is refusing to let this end. My money is being held in court while William delays. So far, this has amounted to a time delay of three years and we have no court date yet. William could have bought the land on completion of the sale of the farmhouse, a year after our divorce. So far he has managed to create a delay of 632 days and counting!

The cost to me in terms of mental health has been a continued severe form of complex PTSD caused by having to constantly relive the abusive life in order to respond to his false claims and present my own witness statements.

You may be exhausted with all of this a good few pages ago and believe me I am too. I am doing my best to be kind to myself and give myself some spoiling on occasions. I find it is no good waiting for this to end before I begin my next journey. After all, it is the journey that counts not the destination. Spending time appreciating what I have every day is a great relief from the daily burden of this divorce.

The cost to me in terms of finance is that I now have legal fees in excess of £..,000, costs of counselling of over £..,000 and a tax bill coming up for the sale of the land of over £..,000. All this is to defend myself in his game. I need a change of game plan!

- *Be pragmatic, yes, but there's being pragmatic and being pragmatic. Don't overdose on pragmatism. You always have to trust yourself and your decisions. When it starts to feel like you have given more than enough, trust your gut. You are an empath and so you always give. Make sure you give to yourself as well and recognise that the difficulties are a result of your abusive ex-partner and not you. Be kind and forgiving to yourself always.*

Remembering the good things

How can I pick you up now that I made you wade through the carnage of our broken relationship? I think the same way I picked myself up. It was an amazing release when I finally left William and realised that I now had a whole new life, which I could lead on my own terms. I wrote down and counted all the good things which had been part of the last twenty years and all the successes I had achieved. This ranged from a successful lettuce-growing season to being part of the group presenting the post-Brexit agricultural policy to the government. I felt so calm once I was alone in a new country with just sunshine and blue sky and peace to heal myself. I could look back in safety and remember the good times and not let them become clouded by the bad ones.

Pandemics and remoteness

Coronavirus 2020 and I am in lockdown on my own and have moments when I feel very sorry for myself. It is good to have all the communications and social media which enable me to easily access my friends, some company and distractions. At times though, I have nights of restless dreams which attempt to drag me back to the past. I hear the pain of others caught in domestic abuse situations who are suffering by the day and wonder what I can do to help. I decided my own helpline and Facebook page might be something which is accessible to some who are cut off from their social groups and need to talk.

The solitude of my lockdown has also helped me focus on the future. I have realised that whatever the future holds for me, the one person I have to spend the rest of my life with is me! And if I'm going to do that peacefully and joyfully, it is an absolute must that I uphold my moral values and beliefs. Part of this will be to ensure that I never again enter into a relationship with a controlling person who thinks of me and everything important in their lives as a monetary value.

Three weeks into lockdown and I make sure I spend time 'chatting' via messages and posts on my Facebook page and the group I started and doing what I can to encourage those I speak to with motivational quotes and positive thoughts. I also think laughter is a great medicine and lets us leave the real world for a moment and get the 'happy drug' fix! It is quite astonishing how many people are going through or have gone through the same scenarios as me.

While dealing with the situation, I didn't recognise or see the 'other' opportunities I could have taken and that is a reflection I can now use to help others. I know now that it was because of my total loss of self-confidence and esteem that I didn't believe

I could have a better life or deserved one. I kept staying in the relationship and trying to make it better! Of course, because that was a target which I could never meet, my life never did become better. Now that I am free of my past and have overcome the challenges of being an independent person and making my own decisions, I realise that my experience might help others see a way forward. It is quite healing for me. I have always loved to help others (probably the worst mistake I made, staying in our marriage for 25 years and trying to make it a good one!). It also gives me a chance to revisit the past and look at what I did that were strengths and what were my weaknesses. I now have the time, space and safety to be able to make changes. This is great as I can live a life using my strengths and learn from the past how to strengthen the weaknesses. (Although being targeted by an abuser is not a weakness. It is being the target of an aggressive man.) I really think that this lockdown has given me a great opportunity. That is a much more exciting idea than the thought that I CAN'T do things.

- *If you're stuck in a similar lockdown, reach out to anyone and everyone. Join support groups and online meet-ups with people who are on the same journey as you. They will have helpful information for you and you will be able to use your empathy skills to help them. Use the time to yourself as an opportunity to rebuild and revitalise yourself. Take up a new interest (albeit online). Draw up a plan for your new life on your own terms.*

At the moment I am a remote parent as I am in Spain and my son is still at university in the UK . (I have started to drop the 'our' son as I now believe that the parenting is solely down to me.) He may be an adult but he will always be my child. At a distance, I can be objective and helpful with some of the challenges he has and he wouldn't be able to come and see me even if I was just down the road because of social distancing.

Connor and I talk and video chat on a regular basis, and I also write my thoughts and send them to him, just as a reminder his Mum is always there for him.

- *If you are unable to see your family friends and loved ones, use the internet and video chat with them. Write 'old fashioned' letters with your love and thoughts in them. You don't need to send them but they will be a physical reminder for you in the future. There are so many sources of support out there, so reach out. (www.trishvalleys.com)*

Therapy horses

So Spain is four weeks into lockdown and much of the population is holding its breath as it appears that the peak has been reached. Some of the construction workers and factory workers start again tomorrow after the deserted streets of Easter and Semana Santa. I have spent a couple of weeks now getting the content together for my website and deciding how I can follow my real passion in the future. My own use of horses and equine-assisted development was a massively empowering step for me. So now, while I am locked down, I am working on a plan to help others and bring horses into their lives. I sincerely hope we will be free to travel for some retreats with these amazing animals very soon. I believe it should be available for everyone, whatever their reasons, to share some time with these amazing souls.

Once I've had enough time, I want to share this with others around me, whatever their circumstances. Many people may be traumatised by the experience of being shut away for weeks and I hope I can help them to unload their fears and anxieties, together with my horses. This will fulfil two of the unmet needs in my life. One is to spend more time doing what I love and being with the horses. The second is to help others, which, although really that is the horses' job, I will be able to facilitate!

The positives of lockdown for me are that I have had a great deal of time I can spend with myself and looking deeply inwards and finding many new strengths. I have appreciated not having to do anything and in fact spending time doing just what I want. I have taken a look at a lot of the 'shoulds' that were in my life and used these few weeks to remove most of them. They do still pop into my thoughts, so as a good measure I have written my success plan and taped it on the kitchen door so that I can read it on a regular basis. It is my idea of success anyway!

- *While you are isolating or locked down, get a plan together for your future. What would you like to do, see or achieve in the next five years? Write it down, and then devise a plan of how you will do it. Two plans! One if lockdown continues and one if it doesn't. Look deeply inwards to find your strengths and desires. Write them all down before you decide which course you will set sail on first.*

My Successful Life as written on my kitchen door!

My success is the freedom to choose where my energy and motivation will flow each day.
I will make a daily choice of how I will succeed and what I really need to do.
I am empowered and have the ability to remove 'shoulds' when they arise.
I will live each day with a smile, much love, joy and inner peace.

- *It is short but that makes it easy to follow and also builds back my self-confidence in believing that I can make excellent choices every day and succeed at them.*

Some of the last nine weeks, while we have been in lockdown, have been quite traumatic. Spain had one of the strictest regimes in the world. It hasn't all been bad, as it has given me a great time to reflect and think about the past. I have reflected on my marriage, and realised that William is probably a narcissist. What has it given me? What can I learn from the experience and use in my future? Strangely, it has been quite a good time for me to do some healing with myself. Don't get me wrong, there were some very bad times and very low points. At those times, I have to thank my son, friends and family for their support which kept me going. I am a little better with my PTSD and I believe that I'm learning not to let the triggers get to me quickly. Take a break, stay in the NOW and sometimes go and suck lemons! I have learnt to do whatever I need to make sure I am quite balanced and calm before responding to any triggers. I am somehow keeping the past where it should always be, in the past. Slowly, I'm time tagging the trauma memories and acknowledging their place in my life. Previously, they have rushed me from behind and I have let myself be engulfed by it. Now I can look back without jumping back into the past. I hope that makes sense.

Another valuable thing I have found by spending time with me alone is I have forgiven myself! I have spent many years beating myself up and my self-talk has been mean and vicious. I wouldn't have said any of the things I was saying to myself to my worst enemy, let alone a friend I love. That's what I am and from now on I'm making it a must to be my own best friend. It's a lovely place to be!

- *Give yourself space and time. Love yourself and be kind. Talk to yourself how you would talk to your best friend if they had these troubles. Forgive yourself and appreciate all that you have. Do this every day whether you are locked down or not.*

Family thoughts

I asked my son for his views on how he dealt with the divorce of his parents. I explained I was writing about this chapter of my life and that I would like him to have his input if he wanted to. There was a bit of breath-holding for a few weeks while he thought about it. One night I asked him if he had time to think about it and we had an hour's chat about the whole experience from his point of view. We didn't discuss his whole life and really only the final stages since I filed for the divorce. At first, he didn't really notice any changes but later found he would have liked more opportunity to access external help and support for his own emotional health and well-being. He thinks that this area of life should be discussed much more broadly in schools and colleges. He believes it would help people recognise these types of abuse and also how to support someone going through similar circumstances. He would like to think that if a light was shed on what is very often hidden outside the home, it may help to reduce it. He also acknowledges that it would be good for children to have an independent source where they can talk and explore the worries and stresses they have over parents divorcing.

I thought Connor's ideas were grounded and measured and that somehow he has found ways of coping with the stress of this. I also recognised that there have been many times when I have been more wrapped up in my own emotions and not necessarily paying attention to his suffering. I hope that going forward Connor can use this experience to make better decisions with his own children.

- *Ask your children for their thoughts and let them express their feelings without fear of any comment or reprisal. Work out with them how you want to be as a family going forward. Promise them you are always there to listen and support them. Don't punish them for loving the parent you are now separated from. That person will always be their parent. If it is a difficult relationship, help them to manage their feelings. You are always the parent and they are your children. Do not expect them to carry the burden of your emotions and trauma.*

New Adventures

My plan for my new future is constantly evolving. I think this is because I am starting to grow and move forward to my new future and I want to be able to put all of this experience to good use to help others. Because of coronavirus, there are many self-help online services appearing. I don't want to be just another one of those. I want to be the coach for those who are reinventing themselves after narcissistic and/or abusive relationships. I want to help them to find themselves and who they want to be and what they want to do in the future. Until I had a clear idea of who I am becoming and where I want to go, I could not plan. So I believe this is critical to helping people define themselves and their future.

I keep telling myself that I am nearer the end of the tunnel than the beginning. It is a good thing I enjoy travelling, because sometimes this route seems to have endless twists and turns. This is a consequence of leaving an abuser and having an expectation that they would be fair, positive and reconciled to a life apart. In my naivety, I imagined that both of us would be able to put aside differences after the divorce and concentrate on co-parenting Connor and do what was in his best interests. My idea of co-parenting and William's differ considerably. For my part, I have spent the last six years doing what I can to protect Connor from the fallout of the divorce. On the other hand, William has got progressively worse in his attempts to use Connor as one of his weapons against me. I believe children have a very difficult time in any divorce and I have always tried to consider the impact of my actions on Connor and reduce it as much as I can. There have been very difficult times when I tried to explain to Connor the reason for our initial separation. He also had some difficulty in recognising that it was nothing to do with him and that he was not in any way responsible or to blame for the divorce. It is never a good time for a divorce and I found choosing the moments to have conversations with Connor very awkward. Many times I felt too emotionally vulnerable to have an objective chat. However, we managed and I believe I quietened Connor's fear that I would never have married if it had not been for his birth.

I believe it would probably have been better to involve Connor at an earlier age, with my thoughts and explanations as to what was going on. However, in hindsight, it is easy to recognise what needed to be done and when. I sincerely hope that I will never get myself into this kind of situation again. Regardless, I will always continue close communication with Connor, whatever the subject is. That way I believe we will be more prepared and able to find coping strategies more quickly with any event or situation.

- *Recognise that when you have made a choice you now want to change, you can. Be accountable. It is not wrong to see things differently with hindsight and to tell others you have had a change of mind. Keep up communication with your children and family and friends. They may not understand what you are going through, but they will appreciate being included in your thoughts. Very often they will have a nugget of wisdom to give you too.*

Making a written record

Since he was born, I have always written a letter to Connor on his birthday and at Christmas. I wanted him to always have a record of his life through my eyes. I wrote it like a sandwich, all good for the first slice, then a slice of what needs to be worked on, and finished with a great slice and optimism for the future. I found that this was also a way that I could give Connor unemotional, factual information. Often when I had spoken to him it gave me a safe way to impart information I thought would be important for him. I remember, just before he went to university he was really upset about our divorce and tried to blame himself. I wondered how many children thought like him. In addition to reassuring him physically and verbally, I wrote to him. I felt it was important to let Connor have something he could always refer to and read for reassurance once he was away at university.

This desire to leave a written record for Connor may have been born out of the fact that I was adopted as a child and had no record of my birth Mum. This was then strengthened by my step-daughters who had lost their Mum at a very young age. I used to hear others say to them that their Mum would have been so proud of them, but they only had these people's word for it, not their Mum's. I was determined that whatever happened in life, Connor would always know what his Mum said and not what someone else thought she would say.

For years, I didn't say anything to Connor about my relationship with his father. I didn't think that it was anything to do with him and didn't want to involve him in our argument. Regrettably, he witnessed some of the arguments and also became the butt of his father's sarcasm and derision over the years before I had applied for the divorce.

His father, as is typical of many abusers and narcissists, always put Connor down and disparaged his talents and abilities, that is, unless he was talking about the fact that he was the father. When William boasted that Connor was amazing, he claimed credit as his father. Never did he ever credit Connor with having earned respect, friends and love on his own merit.

This was an attack on Connor's self-esteem and confidence and I have no doubt it has had an impact. I regret not taking action to protect Connor from this sooner, but

I was in such a low place, I could not get over myself enough to see the bigger picture. The positive of this is that Connor has a much better respect for himself and view of his value to the world. I am very proud of his inner strength and resilience, and hope that he can also use this experience of life to guide himself in a balanced and emotionally stable way through his future.

As an aside, looking back at photos of Connor's life, there are none taken with me after the day of his birth. Every staged family photo is taken by me and is of William and Connor. I am still smarting with the memory of being told all my failings and why I shouldn't be in a photograph at all, let alone with Connor. I am a little sad at this but have realised that life is about creating wonderful memories to look back on, and I believe Connor has many, many such happy memories stored up that were created by his Mum. I spend time painting pictures with regular letters and cards to Connor (in addition to the factual updates) and I believe this is a way to help Connor cement happy memories and time tag the unhappy ones.

I am still not comfortable with being in photos as the bad memories still lurk at times. The saboteur in me still tells me I'm fat, ugly and not worthy. I put these aside now and let it go. I have realised that by doing this and forgiving myself, these memories can't hurt me and allow me to move forward in life. I have painted many pictures with words so that Connor and I both have those in our memories and can enjoy a special way of being together always.

- *Keep the communication going and learn to talk to your children and be open. It is easy with hindsight to know what should have been done differently. Let them know that, but stay accountable, don't hide away from the sadness or the problems. Recognise and acknowledge the bad times and undertake to work hard to ensure that it is not repeated in the future. You are human and life happens. Mistakes are only mistakes if you fail to recognise the learning and keep repeating them.*

Not in the middle

Further to the timeline which I originally gave Connor, I have recently had to do an update. We were having a conversation about the future and finances, when I mentioned that because of the pandemic it was unlikely that the final hearing to settle the money, which is being held in court, would be relisted before 2021.

Connor then mentioned that some three weeks before, on Father's Day, his Dad had defied lockdown restrictions and driven to see him. He had taken with him a file of papers to show Connor (I know not what), and had told Connor that he wanted all the money which was being held by the solicitor for the land, paid to Connor, but I wouldn't agree. However, he also confessed that he was quite happy for all the money to be wasted on legal fees while we waited for the next court hearing. Connor hadn't said anything to me at the time (I suspect his father was hoping for the opposite) but did mention that he was concerned. Once again, I realised my lack of an update had put Connor in a difficult position, caught between William and myself, and only having heard Williams' side of the story. I did another factual timeline starting from the previous letter and demonstrated the delay and prevarication his Dad had caused. It also showed the number of times he had changed his financial statement and repeatedly adding new claims of debts I owed him. Connor had been put in the middle by his father. I felt it only right that he should have the choice of whether the money was paid to him or not. I explained that, for me to be legally and financially free of William, it was not just a question of paying out the money. Total and complete freedom required the dissolution of all the existing farm partnerships, the final tax accounts would need to be agreed upon along with William agreeing to drop all and any future financial claims against me. All of this would have to be agreed upon and would need to coincide with the payment of the money. I had come to realise that in order to have a full and final break from William it was something that would have to be achieved by a court, as all attempts between ourselves had been futile and just led to endless delays and legal costs. William had backtracked on every agreement we had ever made and had only cooperated under pressure from the court. I assured Connor that I was reconciled to waiting for my day in court.

At this moment, Connor has said he will accept the money and so my solicitor has written to William's solicitor with the offer. We have a few more days to wait to see if this is finally the end for me and if William accepts. It is my truly final attempt at trying to resolve this without the need of a judge and the costs involved, but as I have said, I am reconciled to my day in court should William stall again. Now that I recognise the games that abusers play, I think this is just another tactic for William to continue demonstrating his control. Although he is the one who has suggested all the money being paid to Connor, I am not confident that he will actually agree to it. Why would he? It would mean that both Connor and I are no longer obliged to have any connection with him if we don't want to. I can't believe he will give up those ties easily. The learning for me from this most recent action by William is that I have resolved to give Connor factual and financial updates on a much more regular basis so that he is never in a position of not knowing when his father is telling the truth or distorting information. Accepting that all the balance of the monies I should have had as part of our divorce settlement should go to Connor is difficult. I have no problem with my son having the funds, but am now in a very difficult financial position and have to have another review of my life! If I am not careful, it also feels a bit like the coercive control wins and that is what William would want – me with nothing! That may seem rather a grandiose statement, and why should Connor believe my truths? I don't quite mean it like that. I mean that he will have both parties' versions of the facts and so he can perhaps make his own balanced decisions, rather than ones which either William or I want him to make.

All the way through this process, I have spent time on my own self-development and learning ways to not only help me but also Connor. Just lately, I have been reading about the benefits of developing a personal and a family mission statement. I have spoken to Connor about it and we are going to develop something which we can share and use to support our little family as a mutual agreement going forward. Most importantly, we keep our communication going and our relationship thriving.

- *A journal and a timeline of events and facts are valuable. The brain distorts emotional thinking, but when you have facts as evidence, it helps ground you and remember properly. This stops you from enhancing the fear and anxiety. It lists what you have done and achieved in life and gives you a feeling of incredible abundance. It time tags the trauma memories and fixes them in the past. It shows you the many wins you've had and isn't clouded with the traumatic emotional times. It also helps you to present the facts to your children as just information rather than with emotional bias.*

I believe I have amassed great fortunes, as I have the love of a wonderful son and stepdaughters and many family and friends. I have my values intact and the emotional space and freedom to continue being an empath and living life on my own terms.

- *The abuser in your life might rate their wealth in money terms and what they have in the bank and assets. Actually that smacks of poverty.*
- *Readers, let this carry you through, the pain will disappear when you start forward with your new life as the incredibly resilient and wise person you have become.*

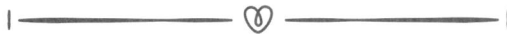

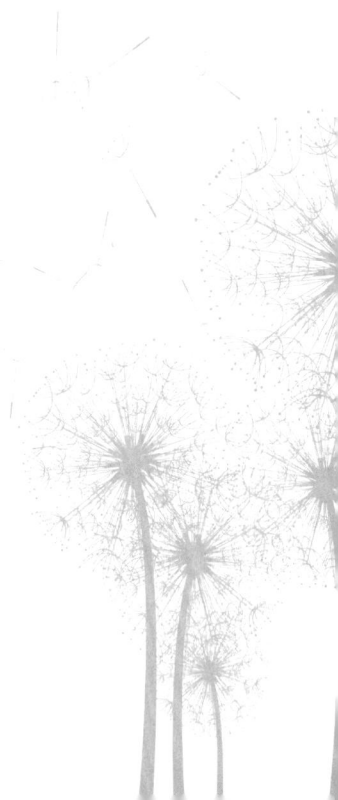

—————— ♡ ——————

Some final thoughts

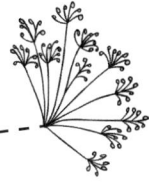

Counting the losses

What I have lost was an illusion of a perfect family that I spent years trying to maintain and convince myself was the truth.

The never being good enough and no self-worth.

Feeling it's all my fault and I have to make it better.

Being treated like an object or valued according to what I have in the bank, rather than for me as a whole person.

Counting Losses as wins

I've lost the feeling that somehow I was a lesser human.

I've lost being berated and put down and belittled every day.

I've lost my lack of confidence.

I've lost being dependent and unable to decide for myself.

I've lost the constant stress and worry and feeling ill and unable to cope.

I've lost the feelings of guilt and shame.

Counting the wins

I've gained self-esteem and independence.

I've gained self-respect and faith in my ability to achieve and be successful in anything I choose.

I've gained inner peace and tranquillity.

I've regained happiness and enjoyment from the simplest things in life.

I've gained my freedom from a life of coercion and abuse.

I've learnt a great deal about myself and grown.

I've learnt to speak out against discrimination and abuse and how shining a light in these dark places must one day be addressed by society.

I'm living life on my own terms.

I've removed the word guilt from my vocabulary.

I'm living the way I want and with myself at peace.

I'm happy and smile a great deal every day.

I'm resilient.

I'm successful.

I hope I've set my son an amazing example.

I believe that the six-plus years and £.,000 to get this far is great value. I have hope and joy and a bright future pulling me forward and each day a sense of a great new adventure.

I feel that I have an unfinished mission. The experiences I have had with institutions (police, the legal system, the estate agents, the property ombudsman the government agencies), all currently uphold and support the behaviour of a manipulative person, albeit unintentionally, and the way policies and tradition operate in many instances.

The project of self-development is a work in progress, but I love my work and the challenges and the journey.

I feel the love and warmth of my family and friends every day.

I have dropped expectations and I spend time appreciating all that I have every day.

I have spent time making myself part of a completely new network of friends This has been exciting and rewarding as I have found many like minds and kindred spirits. Above all, they are empaths like me. I have also got on board with an amazing life coach who pushes me to be the best I can be and holds the mirror while I reflect on all my achievements, and the many wins I have each day. She has helped me on the journey of my new life on my terms.

Another very good friend has just asked me if I am going to remain in Spain return to the UK, or become a global nomad. Global nomad, that really struck a note with me. What does a global nomad look like for me? Where do global nomads travel How exciting and mysterious that future might be. I realise now that wherever my journey takes me, I have all the skills and resources within me to make that journey alone and independently and have great fun along the way. Many people have spoken of the therapeutic value of writing this down and getting it out of my system. would disagree with that view on some levels. While writing I found I was re-living trauma and found that terribly difficult to manage. My coping mechanisms have been comfort-eating and inordinate amounts of alcohol at times. There has been a physical emotional and health impact in getting this story written. Maybe there should be a health warning attached to the reading as well? I hope those readers who have been in the same places in life will not be re-traumatised. Instead, I hope they feel the comfort that there are others in the world who understand and have managed to survive and turn their lives into much happier times. For me, I am now living life on my own term and it is the life I deserve. It is my dream and it is what I want. I feel it is aspirational and a new adventure every day, which fulfils and satisfies me.

- *I want to throw light on the inequality and campaign for all institutions to review and change policies and procedures where needed to function in a more impartial way. Discrimination in any form must be removed from our society. Often it is easily seen because of issues of colour, sex or employment, but very often I think it is overlooked and not considered as inequality. I have a great belief in education. With education, the world can change and I believe we must educate everyone to recognise these hidden and overlooked institutionalised discriminations and take action. At the same time, I want to do my bit to raise more awareness and understanding of a form of violence that often goes unrecognised andin so doing protects the abusers.*

- *I hope you will be inspired to stand up and be accountable. You are a survivor and now it's your time to move on with a new and rewarding life. Channel your focus on you and what you want and where your focus goes, energy flows. A coach or a mentor, whatever you choose to call them, will help you to become whatever you want to be, so push yourselves just because you can! Get a therapist too. I have found my therapy sessions invaluable. They have given me many hours of safe space and guidance to examine some deep-rooted traumas and resolve them and place them in the past where they rightfully belong. I have learnt from David (my coach), that it is much better to confront and examine the issues than try and forget, and have them haunt my days and nights forever! If I never live with anyone else, I will live with myself all the rest of my life. Therefore, it's good if I and myself agree on our values and share the same principles!*

It has been an exhausting trip, but last night I felt very calm and totally at peace. For now, I want to stay in that world. I know that in many ways this story will never be finished because that's not the way for a coercive controller. I have made many edits and no doubt there are many more I should make. However, you will have to accept this as it is because I am not able to muster any more strength right now. I believe some of those reading will have been in the same place and can understand that statement. Maybe, I'll get to writing some more thoughts and maybe you'll join me for the next chapter sometime? Above everything, I want you to know that it is a wonderful place to be at the other end of the tunnel. It is so great feeling that I'm worthy again and that it's ok to stop and take a look around me and enjoy my world just as it is today. It is great to spontaneously laugh and know that I'm not going to be put down or criticised for just being me! It's a feeling that makes me want to run and skip, and I do hope these notes and tips help more of you to get to the same place. See you there I hope!

Acknowledgements

As with most books, this is a collaboration of effort from my family, friends and loved ones. I had the content and they helped me through all the lessons I have learned. It began as my way of helping myself to recover and move forward with a new life. It has been a painful journey at times, but has also helped me remember the many good times there have been. I value all of you for your input and support and encouragement.

To Marianne and Josephine, without them this book would probably not have been written or published. Their mentoring has been so helpful to me. My english teacher would have been proud of what they have helped me accomplish! Both these amazing people were brought to me through the horses. Marianne has an uncanny knack of connecting with me at my darkest moments and offering a supporting hand. Josephine showed me I can make a difference in other people's lives and from her I learnt .

A special thanks to Kristy Lee Hochenberger, who freely gave her time and thoughts to me and wrote my foreword. Her work will help the world and her expertise deserves to be acknowledged not just in the USA but around the globe

Similar thanks to Dr Emma Katz for all her hard work in the field of domestic abuse and coercive control. I found reassurance from reading her work and hope that she too will be recognised as a leader in her field in the UK. Thanks for your review

To my amazing son who is a constant source of love and joy. For him I would do it all again ... differently!

To my daughters who have never left me in the cold and support me daily. I have learnt so many wonderful lessons courtesy of them!

To all my friends and family. Those who have selflessly put their own problems aside to help and support me.

To the counsellors, coaches and mentors who helped me through and particularly Richard who answered my cry for help first. He has spent many expert hours patiently holding the mirror for me so that I could explore my true self and my experiences safely.

To Michelle and Darius for your skills, empathy and untiring support of my efforts at writing.

To special friends Tracey & Simon for never leaving my side, and having a floodlight handy when needed. Another special friend Julic who stood beside me and pointed out the numpties in my life.

June and all those who read my efforts and gave so freely of their feedback.

To my coach Giada whose coaching skills showed me how to love and trust myself again and how to live life on my own terms. Every time I thought I'd reached my limits she was there to give me the nudge I needed to rise to the challenge.

To sleep and all the benefits I felt once I was no longer deprived.

To all the readers of this journal who are on this journey with me. Without you I would not feel I was making a contribution to raising awareness and understanding of domestic and narcissistic abuse and coercive control.

To the amazing horses in my life who have borne the load and ditched my baggage for me in their stoic, easy natural way.

To the friends far and wide who have helped me through and shone the light for me when the tunnels were long and dark

Without all of you I would not be in a position to make a difference.

To me and my new life living it on my own terms. Without facing these demons I would not have been freed and validated!

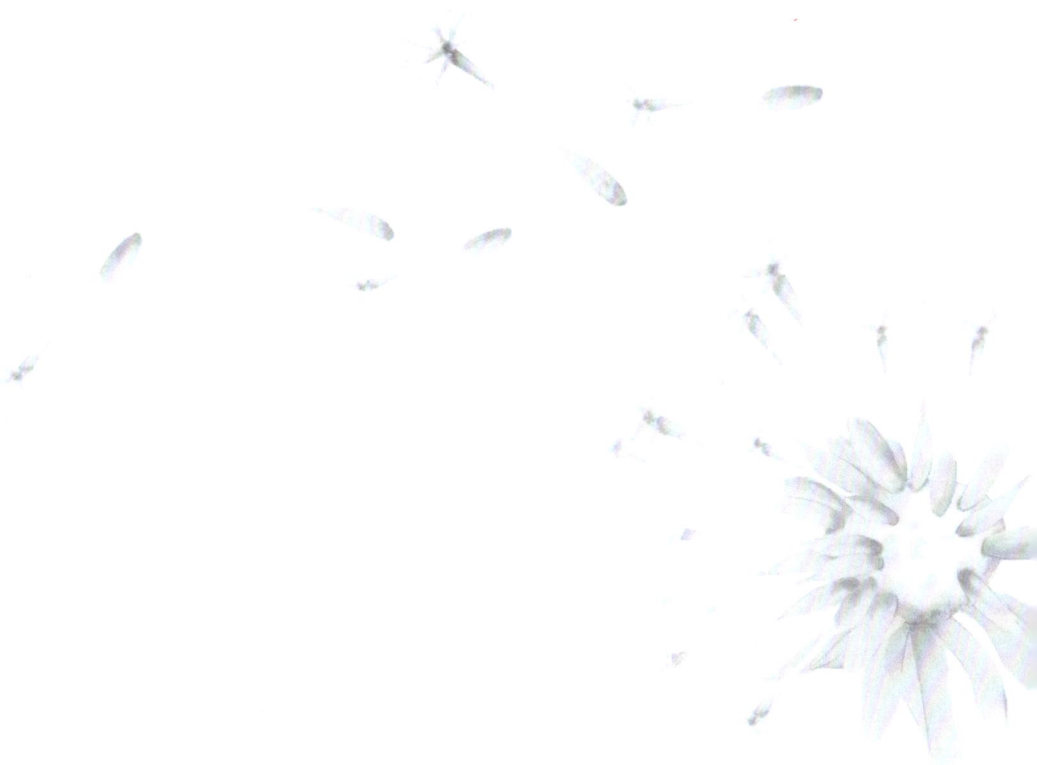

Reviews

I asked a couple of friends to read what I had written and give me feedback and this is what they said.

Hi Trish, Happy new year.

I have spent the whole of this morning reading your book. Trish, you never cease to amaze me, I think it is really the most enormous long and tortuous journey you have been on, over the course of the years I had forgotten or put to the back of my mind some of the wicked details that William subjected you to. I can only say that I think you are the most marvellous person to have come through such an experience and still be so positive about your life and future.

Frankly, torture is not an exaggeration of some of the things he did to you. I think this book is both good for you and for others who are experiencing similar treatment to be put out into the open for examination, too much gets hidden out of shame or a feeling of failure or guilt. BE PROUD OF WHAT YOU HAVE ACHIEVED!!! It is quite shocking that such sexual discrimination still abounds amongst the powers that be and certainly needs highlighting.

Well done lovely girl xx

Hi Trish,

Incredible book,

You went through so much, and what is extraordinary is you didnt loose yourself.

You should be proud of yourself

All the best